Stage 2 – Drug treatment

Drugs must not be given until cardiac massage provides adequate blood flow.
Asystole (commonest in anaesthetised horses)

   Adrenaline IV. Continue massage and IPPV.
     Adrenaline dose 0.3 ml per 100 kg of 1 in 1000 (= 0.003 mg/kg).
If that fails,

   Atropine or glycopyrrolate IV. Continue massage and IPPV.
     Atropine dose: 1.6 ml per 100 kg of 0.6 mg/ml = 0.01 mg/kg.
     Glycopyrrolate dose: 2.5 ml per 100 kg of 0.2 mg/ml = 0.005 mg/kg.
If that fails,

   Adrenaline IV. Continue massage and IPPV.
     Adrenaline dose 0.5 ml per 100 kg of 1 in 000 (= 0.005 mg/kg)

Ventricular fibrillation
   Very unusual in the horse.
   Defibrillate if equipment available.
   Lignocaine IV. Continue massage and IPPV.
     Lignocaine dose: 2.5 ml/100 kg of 20 mg/ml (= 0.5 mg/kg)

Stage 3

Once spontaneous rhythm is restored, treatment depends on the state of the horse as well as the original cause of the problem. Heart rhythm and hypotension may need treatment. If anticholinergics have been used, very small doses of dobutamine should be given or severe tachycardia will occur. Causes of the original arrest, where known should be corrected as far as possible.

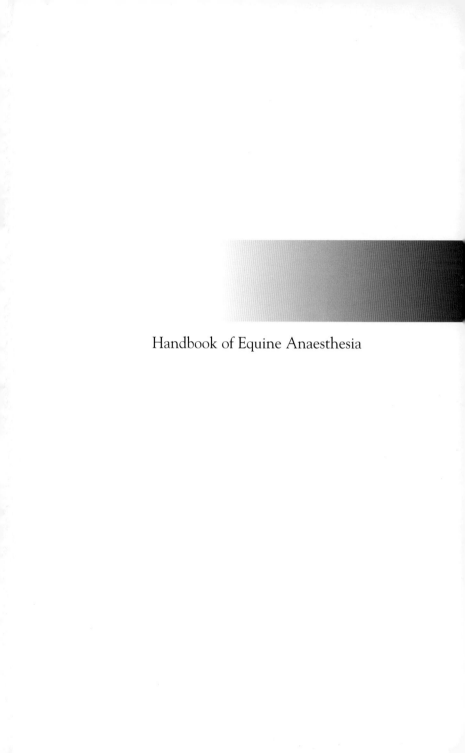

Handbook of Equine Anaesthesia

For Elsevier:
Commissioning Editor: Joyce Rodenhuis
Development Editor: Rita Demetriou-Swanwick
Project Manager: Anne Dickie
Designer: Stewart Larking
Illustrations: Cactus

HANDBOOK OF
Equine
Anaesthesia

Second Edition

PM Taylor
MA Vet MB PhD DVA DiplECVA MRCVS

&

KW Clarke
MA Vet MB DVetMed DVA DiplECVA FRCVS

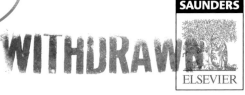

SAUNDERS

ELSEVIER

Edinburgh   London   New York   Oxford   Philadelphia   St Louis   Sydney   Toronto 2007

SAUNDERS
ELSEVIER

An imprint of Elsevier Limited

© Elsevier Limited 2007. All rights reserved.

First published 1999
Second edition 2007

ISBN 10 0 7020 2835 5
ISBN 13 978 0 7020 2835 9

British Library Cataloguing in Publication Data
A catalogue record for this book is available from the British Library

Library of Congress Cataloging in Publication Data
A catalog record for this book is available from the Library of Congress

Notice

Knowledge and best practice in this field are constantly changing. As new research and experience broaden our knowledge, changes in practice, treatment and drug therapy may become necessary or appropriate. Readers are advised to check the most current information provided (i) on procedures featured or (ii) by the manufacturer of each product to be administered, to verify the recommended dose or formula, the method and duration of administration, and contraindications. It is the responsibility of the practitioner, relying on their own experience and knowledge of the patient, to make diagnoses, to determine dosages and the best treatment for each individual patient, and to take all appropriate safety precautions. To the fullest extent of the law, neither the Publisher nor the Authors assume any liability for any injury and/or damage to persons or property arising out or related to any use of the material contained in this book.

The Publisher

Printed in China

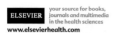
II

CONTENTS

ACKNOWLEDGEMENTS

The authors would like to thank the following clinics where photographs were taken:
The Royal Veterinary College; Cambridge Queens Veterinary School Hospital; The Animal Health Trust; Bell Equine Clinic; Rossdale and Partners; Liverpool University Veterinary School; Dierenkliniek De Bosdreef; New Bolton Centre; and the Veterinary Schools at the Universities of Cornell, Georgia, Colorado and California at Davis.

PREFACE

Smooth and successful equine anaesthesia remains a significant challenge for all those who have to anaesthetise horses - we have had our disasters and near-misses too!

This book is intended for all those who anaesthetise horses; both for those working in a busy surgical clinic as well as for those who do a few procedures per year 'in the field'. The last decade or two has seen considerable progress in our understanding of how the horse responds to anaesthesia. As a result, new techniques, new drugs and new ways of using old drugs have all been employed to allow safer, more controllable anaesthesia in this species. In turn, this has enabled more complex surgery to be undertaken.

We hope that this book will provide a ready reference to state-of-the-art equine anaesthesia. This should enable more horses to benefit from worldwide expertise, experience and advances in this exciting and challenging discipline.

In spite of all the progress with innovative drugs and new methods, the saying 'there are no safe anaesthetics, only safe anaesthetists' remains as true as ever. We hope this book will help produce a few more safe anaesthetists.

The second edition of this handbook has the same intention as the first: to be a real handbook of practical use at the horse's side. We have included new developments in the field, reflecting worldwide expertise and experience. In particular we have included a new chapter on analgesia; probably the most rapidly growing and changing aspect of equine anaesthesia.

P.M. Taylor   **K.W. Clarke**

INTRODUCTION

ANAESTHETIC RISK

General anaesthesia carries a risk of death or serious mishap in any species, but the risk of mortality or serious morbidity is particularly high in horses. The reasons for this are not entirely clear, but probably relate, at least in part, to the effects of the marked cardiorespiratory depression that occurs during anaesthesia in this species. It is essential that the owner of the horse understands that equine anaesthesia carries a significant risk (1% die within 7 days of anaesthesia and surgery) and should sign an indemnity form that states that this is understood. This will not protect the veterinary surgeon against being sued for negligence but will demonstrate that the owner understood the normal risk. If the animal is insured, the insurance company must be informed that it is to undergo anaesthesia and surgery; the information must be given before the procedure takes place, unless it is for emergency treatment. Many insurance companies will not cover death or accidents occurring during anaesthesia unless they have been previously informed that it was to take place.

In addition to the risk to the horse, equine anaesthesia also puts the handlers at risk of injury. Horses are large and potentially dangerous creatures: during induction and recovery, when they may become excited and ataxic, they can all too easily injure a person. Owners and inexperienced onlookers must be kept well out of the way during this period. At least one experienced handler should be present, and the anaesthetist should take overall command during induction and recovery to avoid confusion. Even when a horse appears well sedated it may still respond aggressively to a stimulus; normal precautions about where to stand and how to hold the horse should be taken.

PREANAESTHETIC PREPARATION

PREOPERATIVE ASSESSMENT AND HISTORY

Every horse should undergo a full clinical examination before sedation, and particularly before general anaesthesia. The cardiovascular and respiratory systems are the most important to assess. The aim of the examination is to ensure that the animal is healthy or to detect abnormalities that necessitate special treatment. The history provides the most useful information: is the owner aware of any abnormality, such as inappetance, coughing, nasal discharge, noisy respiration or poor exercise tolerance? Has the horse been sedated or anaesthetised before, and if so, did anything unusual occur? Does it have a history of 'tying up'? How fit is it?

The horse should be examined physically, paying particular attention to general condition and demeanour, the colour of mucous membranes, respiratory pattern and jugular venous filling. The presence or absence of jugular thrombosis should also be noted in order to avoid the subsequent discovery of such thrombosis being attributed to the anaesthetic drugs. The pulse should be palpated and the rate recorded. Any abnormalities such as oedema or multiple enlarged lymph nodes should prompt further investigation. The heart and lungs should be auscultated and any sign of cardiac or pulmonary disease investigated and if necessary treated before elective anaesthesia. In an emergency, anaesthesia will have to be carried out almost regardless of an additional abnormality, but the anaesthetist should be prompted to make special arrangements to compensate for any additional problems. In all cases owners should be informed of any abnormality detected so that they are aware of the increased risk and can decide whether they wish for further investigation or treatment before the horse is anaesthetised.

Respiratory disease

A horse with chronic obstructive pulmonary disease (COPD) should be kept in dust-free conditions and given suitable medical treatment before elective anaesthesia. However, if it is presented for emergency colic surgery it should have oxygen supplied as promptly as possible, both at induction and in the recovery period.

A horse with upper respiratory tract infection or pneumonia should be treated and rendered symptom-free before anaesthesia. There is also the potential for transmission of infection to the next case via contaminated anaesthetic breathing systems. A pneumonic horse requiring colic surgery carries a very high risk.

Cardiac disease

Cardiac murmurs do not necessarily indicate that the horse should not be anaesthetised. If there is no sign of heart failure, exercise tolerance is normal, jugular filling is normal and there is no oedema, anaesthesia can be carried out without additional risk. If there is concern that the condition might be causing symptoms, a cardiac scan can be undertaken.

Cardiac dysrhythmias detected by auscultation must be followed up before anaesthesia. Even a horse with colic should undergo ECG investigation if atrial fibrillation is suspected. Dysrhythmias that affect output, such as atrial fibrillation, should be treated before elective anaesthesia.

Special tests
Special tests such as haematology and biochemistry are unnecessary if the history and clinical examination do not detect any abnormalities. Some prefer to measure at least haematocrit and plasma protein, although it is unlikely that the conduct of the anaesthesia would be altered as a result of any marginal changes that were not suspected from the clinical examination.

Horses presented for emergency surgery carry a higher risk, both because of the disease process itself and because there is less opportunity to investigate any other abnormalities. The special problems of such cases are covered in Chapter 8.

ROUTES OF DRUG ADMINISTRATION
Anaesthesia in horses is usually induced by intravenous (IV) injection. Because the brain has a large blood supply the horse becomes unconscious in the time it takes the drug to move from the site of injection to the brain. This allows the handler to control induction, as it must occur within seconds to a few minutes of injection. Intramuscular (IM) injection is rarely used in horses to induce anaesthesia as the absorption of drugs is slow and variable. IM and IV injections are used for premedication and sedation. However, a slow onset after IM injection is often preferable for premedication and may lead to more consistent sedation and fewer side effects than after IV injection. IM injections carry the risk of local reaction, infection and abscessation, and must be given with full aseptic precautions. Subcutaneous (SC) injections are rarely used for sedation or anaesthesia in the horse. Similarly, with the exception of acepromazine (see page 20), these agents are not usually given by the oral route as onset is slow and unpredictable. Many drugs are either inactivated in the stomach or metabolised in the liver before they can produce an effect. The sublingual route, however, is suitable for drugs such as detomidine (see page 22), which are well absorbed through mucous membrane but are inactivated in the stomach.

IV injections are most commonly given into the jugular vein in horses. This is easy to locate, but in thin-necked horses, foals and small ponies it is easy to hit the carotid artery by mistake. Anaesthetic drugs injected into the carotid artery can be lethal as they are transported straight to the brain. If this occurs the horse 'falls off the needle', as the animal is often affected before the injection is complete. Violent excitement and, commonly, death occur. Great care must be taken to ensure that jugular injections really are intravenous. The colour and rate of flow help to differentiate arterial from venous blood. The needle or catheter should be placed in the vein and the blood allowed to flow out freely before a syringe is attached and any injection is made (Figure 1.1). The use of a small-gauge needle or catheter makes it more difficult to distinguish between arterial and venous puncture. The technique of maintaining the vein in the raised position while the IV injection is made helps to prevent accidental subcutaneous injection.

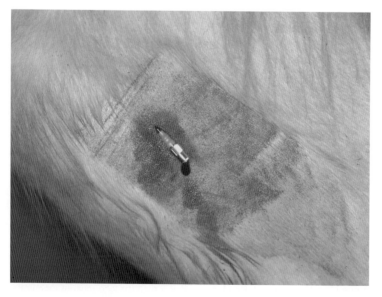

FIG 1.1 The needle or catheter is inserted into the vein and blood allowed to flow out freely before a syringe is attached and any injection made.

However, all the drug is released into the circulation when the pressure is removed, therefore care is needed if the particular drug requires a slow injection.

CATHETERISATION

An IV catheter should always be placed before induction of anaesthesia. Even before short 'field' procedures it is a wise precaution, as it allows additional doses of anaesthetic to be given if the procedure turns out to be more complex than anticipated. It also provides a ready venous access should drugs need to be given in emergency. In major surgery, IV access is also required for fluid administration, for additional drugs and for supplementary IV anaesthetics. Routine use of a catheter prevents both drug wastage and tissue necrosis from inadvertent perivascular injection.

A simple 'over the needle' catheter is placed in a jugular vein under aseptic conditions. It should be sufficiently long (8–12 cm) to prevent it from being dislodged during induction. There is no difficulty in placing large-diameter catheters in horses, and at least 14 standard wire gauge (swg) should be used to allow rapid fluid administration; 16 swg may be used in very small ponies. Catheters can be placed pointing either into the flow (up the neck) or with the flow (down the neck). It is usually easier to place them into the flow, and this position has the advantage that air is not sucked in if the seal is dislodged. However, longer catheters can be used pointing with the flow and it is probably easier to distinguish between arterial and venous blood in this direction, although the risk of air entrainment is increased. Extensions incorporating valves will reduce the chance of air embolism. Even very small volumes of intravenous air can be fatal. The orientation of the catheter appears to make little difference to the induction of anaesthesia or intravenous infusion, although 'with the flow' direction is usually used for rapid infusion of large volumes.

Asepsis is essential during catheter placement. When the catheter is for anaesthesia only a 'no-touch' technique is sufficient, but the skin must be prepared and the operator's hands must be scrupulously clean. In the sick horse, and where the catheter is to remain *in situ* for more than a few hours, full surgical preparation must be used, including sterile gloves.

Catheter placements up and down the vein are illustrated in Figures 1.2a–e and 1.3a–c.

Text continued on p. 10

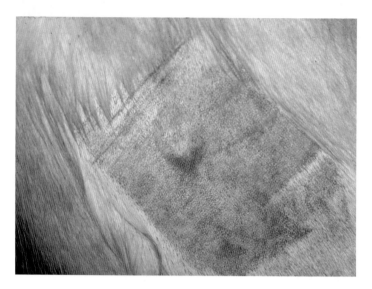

FIG 1.2a Local anaesthetic is infiltrated intradermally with a fine needle until a 1–2 cm diameter weal is raised. A small skin incision may be made into this weal.

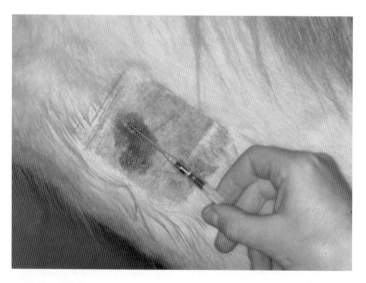

FIG 1.2b An 'over-the-needle' catheter with the needle fully inserted is placed through the skin incision and into the vein at approximately 45° to the skin. In this case the catheter is directed into the flow of blood.

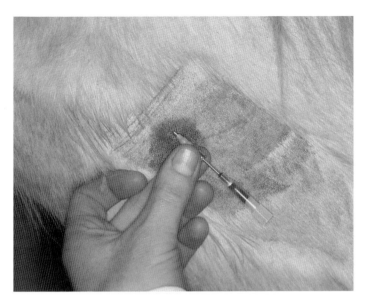

FIG 1.2c A 'flashback' of blood is seen in the catheter chamber and the catheter is advanced off the needle and on into the vein without risk of the needle puncturing the vessel wall.

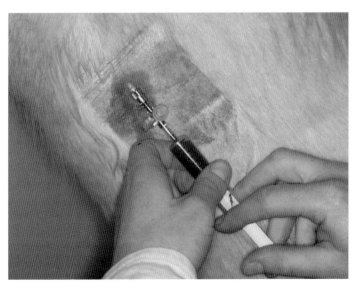

FIG 1.2d A stopcock is attached (an obturator with rubber injection port is also suitable) and the catheter is flushed with heparinised saline (2–10 units/mL).

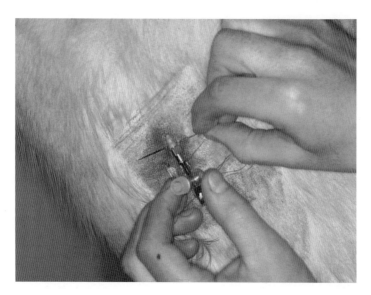

FIG 1.2e The catheter is secured in place with a suture. Alternatively, cyanoacrylate glue can be used.

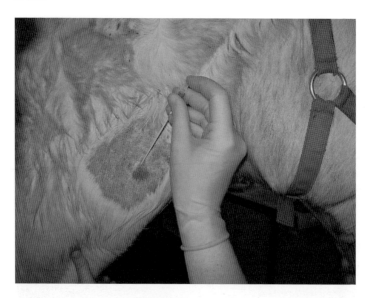

FIG 1.3a After intradermal local anaesthetic and a small skin incision, the catheter is to be placed down the vein. This catheter was to remain in place for more than 24 hours, hence full aseptic precautions, including gloves, are used.

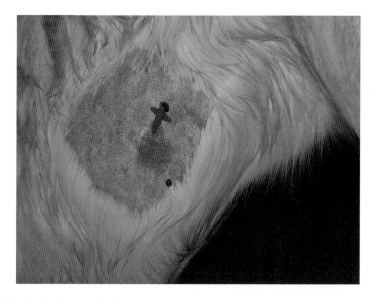

FIG 1.3b Once in place, the vein remains held up with blood flowing specifically to ensure that air is not entrained before the catheter is sealed.

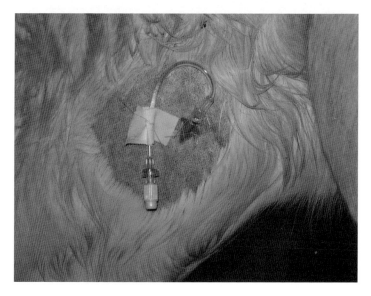

FIG 1.3c An extension incorporating a valve has been attached to the catheter to ensure that air is not entrained. The whole ensemble is stitched in place using a tape 'butterfly'.

WEIGHT

Since most anaesthetic and sedative drugs are given as computed doses, it is essential to have some estimate of the animal's weight. With experience, weight can usually be estimated fairly accurately, but the only way to gain the experience is to weigh a large number of horses.

Purpose-built equine scales are ideal but are only available in larger clinics (Figure 1.4).

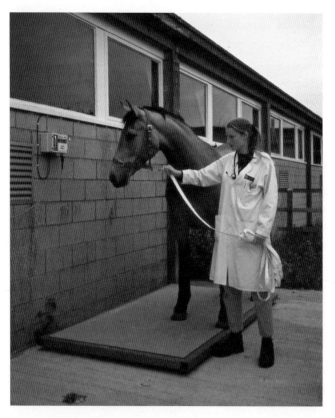

FIG 1.4 *Body weight is best determined with commercial equine scales. Estimates should always be compared with accurate weighing whenever possible in order to develop and maintain the skill.*

Tapes. Fairly accurate estimations can be made with tapes (usually supplied with anthelmintics or from saddlers) marked with weight rather than length. These are placed around the girth or the widest part of the abdomen (according to the manufacturer's instruction) (Figure 1.5). They are not accurate in small ponies, donkeys and foals.

Formula $\text{weight (kg)} = \dfrac{\text{girth (cm)}^2 \times \text{length (cm)}}{10\,815}$

Girth = girth line where saddle is placed
Length = distance from point of shoulder to point of ischium.
This is better than tapes but is still inaccurate in donkeys and foals.

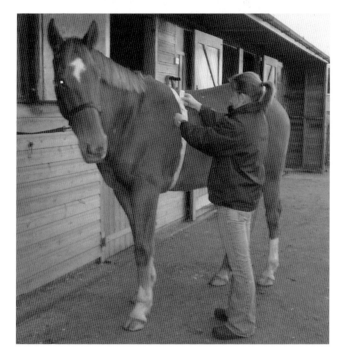

FIG 1.5 *'Weigh tapes' are available from pharmaceutical companies supplying anthelmintics. The horse is measured around the girth and the weight is read from the tape. This provides a good estimate of weight in adult horses and ponies.*

ENVIRONMENT

Equine anaesthesia should not be undertaken lightly, as many things can go wrong. The environment in which the procedure is carried out, from induction all the way through to recovery, must be appropriate. It is quite acceptable to carry out 'field' anaesthesia for short procedures on the premises where the horse is kept (see pages 45–47), but major surgery requires a more sophisticated arrangement. As far as the horse is concerned, induction and recovery must take place in a safe environment. When major surgery is to be carried out on a regular basis this necessitates the use of a padded box. This should not be too large (3 × 3 m is large enough even for Shire horses); it must be solidly constructed (a recovering horse can exert enormous forces on the wall and doors) and have suitable flooring and padded walls (Figure 1.6).

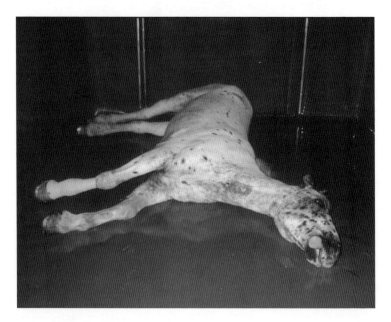

FIG 1.6   A padded recovery box reduces the risk of self-inflicted injury during recovery. A box no larger than 3 × 3 m is small enough to prevent most horses from gaining much momentum. The surface should be padded and non-slip, but easy to clean.

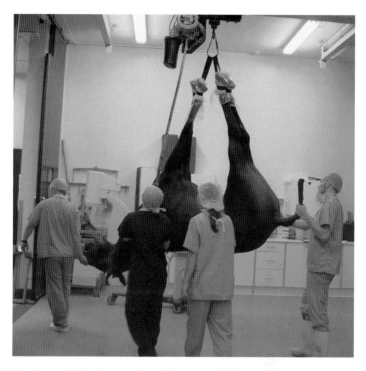

FIG 1.7 *Purpose-built equine operating tables are essential for regular major surgery. The horse must be lifted on and off the table; this is most easily achieved by hoisting the hobbled horse. Other methods, such as a table that forms part of the induction box floor, are used, but the illustrated system is the most simple and versatile*

Some means of lifting the horse on to a table or deep matting is also required. A hoist and purpose-built operating table is ideal (Figure 1.7), but as far as the horse is concerned, as long as it is adequately padded the ground can be used; a table improves the surgeon's comfort.

In addition to a suitable venue, a certain amount of basic equipment is essential for general anaesthesia in horses. Where major surgery is to be carried out on a regular basis it is essential to have a large-animal anaesthetic machine with oxygen supply, a precision out-of-circuit vaporiser, a rebreathing circuit and a range of endotracheal tubes (see Chapter 4). Basic monitoring equipment, such as at least a means of direct arterial blood pressure measurement and an electrocardiograph (ECG) (see Chapter 5), should also be available; capnography is desirable. Although a ventilator is not essential for administering halothane, intermittent positive-pressure ventilation (IPPV) is required more often when isoflurane is used. A ventilator is highly recommended for clinics where large numbers of horses are anaesthetised, whether by inhalation or by total intravenous methods. Some procedures cannot be performed without a ventilator, and many are greatly facilitated with one.

If in doubt, it is far better to refer a horse to a centre that is experienced and has appropriate equipment than to attempt an untried procedure with inadequate facilities.

THE HORSE AS A FOOD ANIMAL

European law, and to some extent in that in most other countries, restricts the administration of any drug to only those licensed in the species in question. In Europe, if there is no appropriate authorised veterinary medicinal product the clinician may treat the animal using the 'cascade':

Schedule 4 Regulation 8 of the UK Veterinary Medicines Regulations (2006) states as follow:

2. (1) If there is no authorised veterinary medicinal product in the United Kingdom for a condition the veterinary surgeon responsible for the animal may, in particular to avoid unacceptable suffering, treat the animals concerned with the following ('the cascade'), cascaded in the following order: (a) a veterinary medicinal product authorised in the United Kingdom for use with another animal species, or for another condition in the same species; or (b) if and only if there is no such product that is suitable, either

(i) a medicinal product authorised in the United Kingdom for human use;

(ii) a veterinary medicinal product not authorised in the United Kingdom but authorized in another member State for use with any animal species (in the case of a food producing animal, it must be a food-producing species);

In the UK, the Veterinary Medicines Directorate has made it clear that it has no intention of interfering with a veterinary surgeon's clinical judgement. Definitive interpretation of the legislation can only be given by the courts.

If carried out to the letter, the legislation makes a mockery of modern veterinary anaesthesia. Numerous 'unlicensed' (i.e. no market authorisation for the species) drugs are essential for safe, controlled equine anaesthesia. A further complication is that European Union legislation designates the horse as a food animal. As a result, the use of drugs in this species should be restricted to only those licensed for use in horses. With the advent of a passport system for horses it is possible for a horse to be designated as a non-food animal, in which case the full cascade applies, and the requirements pertaining to food animals do not apply. Currently, the European Commission is considering allowing a specified list of commonly used drugs that do not have market authorisation for horses (e.g. diazepam, dobutamine) to be used in this species, with a 6-month withdrawal period before the animal goes for human consumption. At the time of writing no final decision has been made, and the list is out for consultation (see Appendix).

In the USA, under the Animal Medicinal Drug Use Clarification Act 1994, the veterinary profession is permitted to use 'off-label' drugs, i.e. those not licensed for use in horses, unless specifically banned. Withdrawal times recommended by the Food Animal Residue Avoidance Data Bank must be adhered to whenever the animal is intended for human consumption.

At present, at least in the UK and the USA, the use of drugs without market authorisation for horses (using the cascade in Europe) is legal if the animals are not to be used for human consumption. However, it is important to appreciate that the efficacy and safety of such drugs in this species have not been legally proven, and the manufacturers are under no obligation to support a veterinary surgeon who has had a problem after using such drugs. Nevertheless, many 'unlicensed' drugs are used on a regular basis.

Further reading

Dean S (2005) Veterinary Medicines Regulations 2005. *Veterinary Record* **157**: 603–605.

Hall LW, Clarke KW and Trim CM (2001) *Veterinary Anaesthesia*, 10th edn. WB Saunders, London.

Johnston GM, Eastment JK, Taylor PM and Wood JLN (2002) The confidential enquiry of perioperative equine fatalities (CEPEF-1): mortality results of phases 1 and 2. *Veterinary Anaesthesia and Analgesia* **29**: 159–170.

Muir WW and Hubbell JAE (eds) (1991) *Muir and Hubbell's Equine Anaesthesia: Monitoring and Emergency Therapy*. Mosby Year Book, St Louis.

Thurmon JC, Tranquilli WJ and Benson GJ (1996) *Lumb and Jones' Veterinary Anaesthesia*, 3rd edn. Williams & Wilkins, Baltimore, 5–34.

2

SEDATION AND PREMEDICATION

There are numerous occasions in equine clinical work when sedation is required for minor surgery or diagnostic procedures. Most of the sedative agents are also suitable for premedication or for use in anaesthetic combinations. The aim of sedation is that the horse should remain standing, and although slight ataxia is acceptable, a motionless horse is the ideal. The horse should be indifferent to its surroundings and should not be aroused by noise, touch, handling or movement (Figure 2.1). Opioid analgesics have long been used to enhance the effect of many sedatives, even in pain-free horses. However, analgesics alone will often calm a horse that is already in pain (see Chapter 6). Whatever sedative is used, the horse should still be handled sensibly as there is always the chance of an unexpected response.

The aims of anaesthetic premedication are to calm the animal, improve the quality of anaesthetic induction and maintenance, reduce the amount of anaesthetic agent used subsequently, and counteract unwanted side effects. Classically, this has been achieved by the administration of sedatives, analgesics and other agents, so that their effects are fully developed before anaesthesia is induced. However, many of the same 'premedicant' agents are now given immediately before, together with, or immediately after the anaesthetic induction agents, as part of an 'anaesthetic combination'. Drugs that cause muscle weakness (e.g. benzodiazepines, guaiphenesin) are most commonly given as part of such a combination.

All sedatives work best when given in a quiet environment. None will produce its maximum effect if the horse is disturbed during or immediately after injection, and so efforts made to keep the environment peaceful are extremely worthwhile. Adequate time must also be allowed for the sedative to have maximal effect. With most sedatives except acepromazine this is reached around 5 minutes after IV injection, but at least 20–30 minutes are required after IM injection. Sedatives and sedative combinations have limited effects; even when they have been used correctly, and even when all suitable precautions have been taken, sedation may not be adequate. When this happens it is necessary to proceed to general anaesthesia. If so, care must be

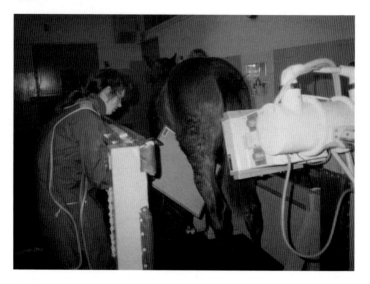

FIG 2.1 Many diagnostic procedures require a still horse, indifferent to its surroundings. For radiography of the limbs sedation must be reliable for the safety of both horse and equipment, as well as in order to produce good films.

taken to allow for the effects of the agents already used on the subsequent anaesthetic protocol.

All drugs used for sedation cause CNS depression and may cause respiratory and cardiac depression. Although this is extremely rare in the sedated horse it must always be regarded as a potential hazard. It is preferable not to move a sedated horse if ataxic, and the sedative is best given where the procedure is to be carried out. No attempt should be made to move the horse until the ataxia has abated. Horses usually remain standing when sedated, but occasionally a heavily sedated horse may fall or lie down. Adequate cardiovascular and respiratory function must be confirmed and the horse should be allowed to remain quiet until ready to stand; it must be allowed space to get up. Where appropriate, antagonists may be given (page 23).

SEDATIVE AGENTS

PHENOTHIAZINES

Of the many phenothiazines available, acepromazine is the most widely used throughout the world. When used on its own, even at low doses, it produces mild tranquillisation and anxiolysis (Figure 2.2). Increasing the dose does little to deepen the sedation. A horse may appear well sedated but still respond when stimulated. Acepromazine is very effective in calming a nervous horse without causing drowsiness or ataxia. Other phenothiazines, such as proprionyl promazine, are used in Europe and their effects are essentially similar to those of acepromazine.

Acepromazine blocks α_1-adrenergic transmission, which is responsible for maintaining vascular tone. It causes blood pressure to decrease, and this may be severe in the hypovolaemic horse. In normovolaemic horses the effect is clinically unimportant. The drug invariably causes penile prolapse lasting a few hours (Figure 2.3). The effect is rarely prolonged. Very occasionally phenothiazines may cause priapism (see Figure 3.9). In either case (prolonged penile

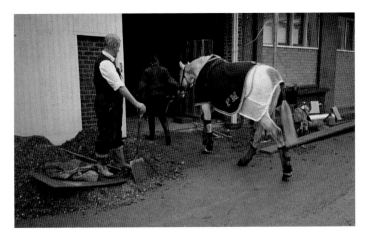

FIG 2.2 *Acepromazine produces mild sedation, anxiolysis and calming with little ataxia. This horse was willing to walk quietly past a noisy building site.*

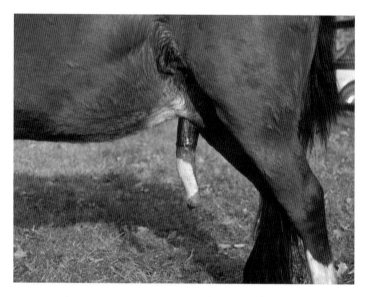

FIG 2.3 Acepromazine causes penile prolapse. The penis must be protected from injury until the effect of the drug wears off.

prolapse or priapism) it is most important that the penis is protected from trauma, or paraphimosis and irreparable damage may occur. As a result of this possibility, the manufacturers of acepromazine contraindicate its use in breeding stallions. However, most anaesthetists consider that it can be used at low doses, provided that immediate treatment is given if this rare complication occurs.

Sedation

Acepromazine is best used at doses of 0.01–0.1 mg/kg, which lasts several hours. It is commonly used at 0.03–0.04 mg/kg. The onset of action is slow: even after IV injection the peak effect is not seen for 15–20 minutes. Oral preparations may also be used, with a maximum recommended dose, as for injection, of 0.1 mg/kg.

Acepromazine is useful on its own in a nervous but otherwise good-tempered horse. It is best for non-painful procedures such as loading, shoeing and sometimes clipping, and an advantage is that the horse often learns to tolerate the procedure. For greater chemical restraint acepromazine is more useful in combination with other agents (Table 2.1, page 29).

Premedication

Acepromazine is an extremely valuable premedicant before general anaesthesia. Although the dose of intravenous induction agents is not greatly reduced, the whole process of induction, and probably also of recovery, is smoothed out. It is particularly valuable in a nervous horse. Acepromazine has been shown to reduce the risk of cardiac arrest in anaesthetised horses. This may be a result of the benefit to cardiac function of the afterload reduction produced by α_1-adrenergic receptor blockade. Alternatively, the protective effect against the development of ventricular dysrhythmias may be important. The only contraindication to the use of acepromazine for premedication is in the hypovolaemic patient, where it may cause severe hypotension.

α_2-ADRENOCEPTOR AGONIST AGENTS: XYLAZINE, DETOMIDINE AND ROMIFIDINE

α_2-Adrenoceptor agonists (α_2 agonists) are used primarily for their sedative properties, but also as analgesics. They produce profound sedation, which reaches its maximum effect within a few minutes of IV administration. The horse adopts a wide-based stance with its head lowered and is apparently oblivious to external stimulation (Figure 2.4). All doses produce ataxia; this is marked after high doses of detomidine and xylazine, but is considerably less with romifidine.

All the α_2 agonists cause a substantial but transient rise in arterial blood pressure and marked bradycardia. Heart rate remains below normal for over half an hour, cardiac output is decreased and respiration slightly depressed. Blood pressure is reduced in the latter stages of sedation. Gastrointestinal motility is reduced and the horse usually urinates copiously. Sweating sometimes occurs as sedation wanes, the incidence being dependent on the length of the horse's coat and on the ambient temperature. The duration of both sedation and of side effects is dose dependent, but xylazine is the shortest acting and romifidine the longest. Additional treatment with anticholinergic vagolytics reduces the bradycardia but hypertension is enhanced; the overall effect on the cardiovascular system is not benefited. One occasional frightening side effect is tachypnoea: the horse 'puffs' for no apparent reason. This appears to be self-limiting and treatment is not required.

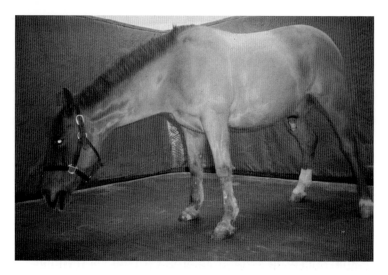

FIG 2.4 α_2-Agonist sedation is profound. This horse has received 0.02 mg/kg detomidine and adopts a classic wide-based stance with lowered head. The effect of xylazine is similar. After romifidine the head is usually not so low.

Sedation

IV injection of 0.5 mg/kg xylazine, 0.01 mg/kg detomidine and 0.05 mg/kg romifidine are satisfactory for many clinical procedures, but more profound sedation is seen with 1 mg/kg xylazine, 0.02 mg/kg detomidine and 0.12 mg/kg romifidine. Maximal sedation is achieved in about 5 minutes. Higher doses (e.g. up to 0.08 mg/kg detomidine) result in increased duration of effects. All the drugs can be given IM, and this route can provide excellent sedation, with reduced severity of some side effects. However, the onset of maximal sedation takes 30–40 minutes and higher than IV doses are required (twice the IV dose of detomidine and three times the IV dose of xylazine). Sublingual detomidine (0.02 mg/kg) produces effects similar to those of 0.01 mg/kg IV, but these drugs have no effect if given orally. Very small doses of detomidine (<0.005 mg/kg) are anxiolytic even if there are no obvious signs of sedation.

The α_2 agonists are used to sedate horses for a variety of clinical diagnostic procedures, such as radiography, endoscopy, clipping and minor surgery under local anaesthesia. Practically, the analgesic properties are more useful for viscera rather than skeletal tissues, and are useful to facilitate the examination of a horse with colic. Small doses give a short period of respite sufficient for procedures such as examination per rectum, but their influence in reducing gut motility must be taken into account and they must be used with extreme care in the compromised horse (pages 185–189).

Horses may appear very heavily sedated under α_2 agonists, particularly detomidine and xylazine, but can kick accurately if appropriately stimulated (e.g. by touch). Increasing the dose of the agonist does not usually improve this effect and a more satisfactory approach is to supplement the α_2 agonist with opioids (pages 26–27).

Antagonists such as atipamezole (0.05-0.15 mg/kg, or 3–10 times a dose of detomidine), although they only carry marketing authorisation for small animal use, have been used successfully to reverse excessive sedation and ataxia that have resulted from accidental overdose.

Detomidine infusion

Detomidine infusions are commonly used to produce consistent sedation over a period of several hours for standing surgical procedures, particularly laparoscopy. The horse is initially sedated with detomidine 0.01–0.02 mg/kg and an opioid such as butorphanol 0.02 mg/kg, and then detomidine alone is infused IV to effect, approximately 0.1–0.2 µg/kg/min, although higher doses may be used at the start. Commonly, 10–20 mg (1–2 mL of a 1% solution) detomidine are added to 500 mL saline, and this is given at up to 10 mL/min in the average 500 kg horse; maintenance is usually around 3–4 mL/min).

Premedication

All the α_2 agonists are used for premedication before induction of anaesthesia with ketamine (page 34) or with barbiturates, where they enable the induction dose to be reduced by up to half (page 41). The undesirable effects on the cardiovascular system may enhance those of anaesthetic agents used concurrently, and in horses with pre-existing disease the doses should be reduced; other premedicant agents may be preferable. However, the advantages of the α_2-adrenoceptor agonists, particularly in ensuring a calm anaesthetic induction, are such that it is rare for them not to be included in an anaesthetic protocol.

BENZODIAZEPINES: DIAZEPAM, MIDAZOLAM, ZOLAZEPAM AND CLIMAZOLAM

Benzodiazepines are not used for sedation in adult horses as they cause muscle weakness and ataxia. However, they are extremely effective for sedation of young foals, which become recumbent so that ataxia is not a problem. Nevertheless, benzodiazepines, generally diazepam and midazolam to are widely used in drug combinations for induction of anaesthesia (Chapter 3) as they cause little cardiovascular depression, although they may enhance respiratory effects. They are potent centrally acting muscle relaxants and are commonly used in combination with the dissociative anaesthetics, where they counteract the increased muscle tone (pages 33–34). They are also valuable as an adjunct to anaesthesia in sick animals.

Benzodiazepine antagonists such a sarmazenil and flumazanil have been used to reverse residual muscle weakness at the termination of anaesthesia.

Diazepam is not water soluble and is generally used in a propylene glycol preparation. A lipid emulsion formulation is also available, but death has occasionally occurred when this formulation has been used for induction of anaesthesia. The cause is unknown.

IV doses of 0.1–0.2 mg/kg diazepam or midazolam produce good sedation in young foals. They usually lie down and will accept a range of non-painful manipulations, such as radiography (Figure 2.5). If anaesthesia is necessary it can then be induced with ketamine (pages 199–200). In adult horses benzodiazepines may be used as part of anaesthetic combinations (pages 36–37 and Table 3.1).

OPIOIDS

The opioids are used primarily for their analgesic properties, and are described in more detail in this context in Chapter 6 (pages 107–110). They are, however, widely used in combination with sedatives to produce profound sedation. In general, opioids cause little sedation in the horse when used on their own, but produce excellent results in combination with small doses of sedatives. Side effects are rarely a problem when used in this way. Butorphanol 0.02 mg/kg, methadone 0.05–0.1 mg/kg, buprenorphine 0.006 mg/kg and morphine 0.1 mg/kg have all been used in combination with sedatives (Table 2.1).

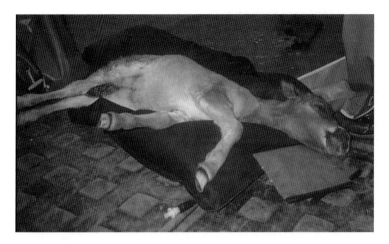

FIG 2.5   Young foals can be sedated with diazepam alone. This foal, less than 7 days old, is recumbent and unresisting throughout extensive radiographic examination.

Premedication

A horse awaiting surgery for a painful condition should have an analgesic included in the premedication. Opioid pain relief will reduce agitation as well as enhancing the effect of any sedative. Horses being prepared for colic surgery are more likely to have α_2-agonist analgesia, but opioid premedication is appropriate prior to orthopaedic surgery. This may enhance ataxia, so a fractured limb should be well supported and the horse should not be required to move (Figure 2.6). An opioid in combination with acepromazine and α_2-agonist premedication is successful (Table 2.1).

DRUG COMBINATIONS FOR SEDATION AND PREMEDICATION

Combinations of more than one sedative are often synergistic and produce better sedation than any one of the drugs used on its own. The use of small doses of two or more chemically different drugs to produce one effect is

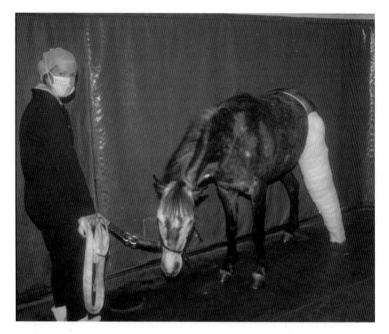

FIG 2.6 An analgesic component should be included in the premedication when a painful condition is awaiting treatment. This pony with a fractured tibia was given flunixin, butorphanol, acepromazine and a small dose of detomidine. In conjunction with good support of the injured limb the result is a calm and relaxed patient ready for induction of anaesthesia.

attractive because the dose of each is reduced. If the two drugs are eliminated from the body by different routes, the chances of toxic effects due to either drug is reduced. Excessive CNS depression, with its concurrent effect on the cardiovascular and respiratory systems, is a potential hazard of combinations of tranquillisers and sedatives. If sensible doses are used this is not a clinical problem.

α_2-AGONIST AND OPIATE COMBINATIONS

The inclusion of an opioid with α_2 agonists produces profound and predictable sedation in standing horses; they are much less likely to kick in

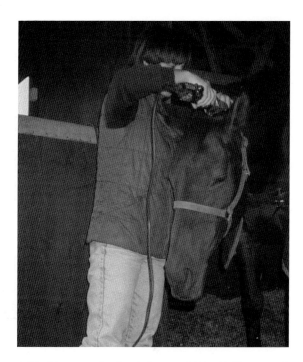

FIG 2.7 *Even the most difficult horses can be clipped when an opioid is added to α_2-agonist sedation. This horse was head shy and detomidine alone was insufficient. Butorphanol and detomidine have produced ideal conditions to clip the head.*

response to noxious stimulation or manipulation than when the α_2 agonist is used alone (Table 2.1; Figures 2.7, 2.8). Whereas α_2 agonists on their own very rarely cause recumbency, even at high doses, overdoses of opioid combinations are more likely to do so.

ACEPROMAZINE COMBINATIONS

Acepromazine is used with α_2 agonists to enhance sedation without causing the profound effect seen with opioids. Some authorities have questioned such combinations, but at the doses recommended (Table 2.1) they have proved safe and efficacious in several thousand horses. The combinations are particularly useful if the horse is frightened or excited prior to sedation,

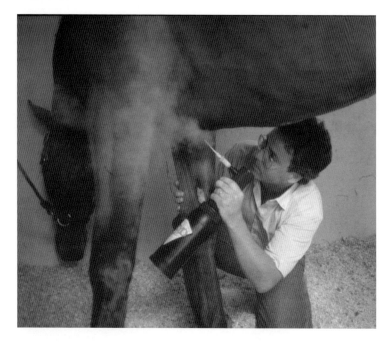

FIG 2.8 Detomidine and butorphanol produce sufficient sedation and analgesia to allow cryosurgery of sarcoids.

although adequate time (up to 30 minutes) may be needed for full effect. Acepromazine can also be included in the α_2-agonist–opioid combination. This increases the degree of sedation and smoothes the return of normal consciousness.

SEDATION (SEE TABLE 2.1)

PREMEDICATION

Sedative combinations, particularly those incorporating the opioids, are used for premedication. Opioids may enhance anaesthetic-induced respiratory depression, but the main advantage is the additional degree of sedation achieved, a calm horse and a smooth induction. Suitable doses are shown in Table 2.1.

Table 2.1 Drug combinations for sedation and premedication

Sedative combination	Dose for sedation	Dose for premedication
Acepromazine	0.02–0.05 mg/kg	0.03–0.04 mg/kg
Xylazine	0.5–0.6 mg/kg	1.0 mg/kg
Acepromazine	0.03–0.04 mg/kg	0.03–0.04 mg/kg
Detomidine	0.01 mg/kg	0.01–0.02 mg/kg
Acepromazine	0.03–0.04 mg/kg	0.03–0.04 mg/kg
Romifidine	0.05 mg/kg	0.1 mg/kg
Acepromazine	0.02–0.05 mg/kg	0.03–0.05 mg/kg
Butorphanol	0.02–0.04 mg/kg	0.02 mg/kg
Acepromazine	0.05–0.1 mg/kg	0.03–0.04 mg/kg
Methadone	0.1 mg/kg	0.1 mg/kg
Xylazine	0.5–1.0 mg/kg	0.5–1.0 mg/kg
Butorphanol	0.02 mg/kg	0.01–0.02 mg/kg
Detomidine	0.01–0.015 mg/kg	0.02 mg/kg
Butorphanol	0.02 mg/kg	0.02 mg/kg
Romifidine	0.05 mg/kg	0.05–0.1 mg/kg
Butorphanol	0.02–0.03 mg/kg	0.02 mg/kg
Xylazine	0.5 mg/kg	0.5–1.0 mg/kg
Methadone	0.1 mg/kg	0.1 mg/kg
Detomidine	0.01–0.015 mg/kg	0.01–0.02 mg/kg
Methadone	0.1 mg/kg	0.1 mg/kg
Acepromazine	0.03–0.06 mg/kg	0.03–0.04 mg/kg
Butorphanol	0.01–0.02 mg/kg	0.02 mg/kg
Detomidine	0.01–0.015 mg/kg	0.015 mg/kg
Acepromazine	0.04–0.06 mg/kg	0.03–0.04 mg/kg
Methadone	0.05–0.1 mg/kg	0.05 mg/kg
Detomidine	0.01–0.015 mg/kg	0.015 mg/kg
Buprenorphine	0.006 mg/kg	
Detomidine	0.01–0.015 mg/kg	

OTHER AGENTS USED AS PREMEDICANTS OR IN ANAESTHETIC COMBINATIONS

ANTICHOLINERGIC DRUGS: ATROPINE, GLYCOPYRROLATE

Use of atropine (0.005–0.02 mg/kg) or glycopyrrolate (0.005–0.01 mg/kg) for premedication in the horse is controversial. Most anaesthetists do not use them routinely but administer them intraoperatively to treat severe bradycardia or to prevent anticipated vagal reflexes (page 192). When given IV they take up to 5 minutes to be effective, and atropine may cause bradycardia before heart rate increases. They reduce intestinal motility and the use of high doses may result in postoperative impaction colic. Hyoscine may also be suitable (page 131).

GUAIPHENESIN

This drug is a centrally acting muscle relaxant that acts at a spinal level; it is used to smooth induction of anaesthesia. It is not a sedative or an analgesic, although it has some hypnotic effects. It affects limb muscles more than respiratory muscles and will induce recumbency without apnoea. It is generally used to induce muscle relaxation in combination with IV induction of anaesthesia using low doses of intravenous agents. On no account should it be used alone for surgery. The solution is irritant and must be given through an IV catheter in as low a concentration as the required volume allows. A 5% or 10% solution is usual; 15% has been used, but higher concentrations cause haemolysis and may damage the intima of the vein. Damage increases with increasing concentration or with too rapid administration, such as that achieved by infusing the drug under pressure.

Clinical use

The guaiphenesin solution is infused until the horse shows signs of ataxia, and anaesthesia is induced with an intravenous agent (Chapter 3). Alternatively, the anaesthetic may be mixed with the guaiphenesin, but this makes it more difficult to judge when the horse will go down. Recumbency can be induced with doses of 100–150 mg/kg guaiphenesin alone, but although it is probably preferable to casting a conscious horse with ropes, this must still be unpleasant for the animal. Guaiphenesin has also been used (up to 30 mg/kg) to produce a degree of muscle relaxation for management of dystocia.

Further reading

Hainisch EK (2001) Sedation by continuous intravenous detomidine drip for standing surgical procedures. *Equine Veterinary Education* **13**: 43–44.

Hall LW, Clarke KW and Trim CM (2001) *Veterinary Anaesthesia*, 10th edn. WB Saunders, London.

Muir WW and Hubbell JAE (eds) (1991) *Muir and Hubbell's Equine Anaesthesia: Monitoring and Emergency Therapy*. Mosby Year Book, St Louis, 247–280.

Thurmon JC, Tranquilli WJ and Benson GJ (1996) *Lumb and Jones' Veterinary Anaesthesia*, 3rd edn. Williams & Wilkins, Baltimore, 183–209.

van Dijk P, Lankveld DP, Rijkenhuizen AB, et al (2003) Hormonal, metabolic and physiological effects of laparoscopic surgery using a detomidine–buprenorphine combination in standing horses. *Veterinary Anaesthesia and Analgesia* **30**: 72–80.

Wilson DV, Bohart GV, Evans AT, et al (2002) Retrospective analysis of detomidine infusion for standing chemical restraint in 51 horses. *Veterinary Anaesthesia and Analgesia* **29**: 54–57.

INTRAVENOUS ANAESTHESIA

In adult horses, anaesthesia is virtually always induced with an intravenous agent. Thereafter anaesthesia may be maintained for short periods with incremental doses of induction agents or, for major surgery, volatile agents are used. In general, the same techniques are used for induction whether anaesthesia is for a short 'field procedure' or before maintenance with inhalation anaesthesia. It is most common to give a computed dose of intravenous anaesthetic agent to induce anaesthesia in horses. It is difficult to 'give to effect' to a large animal that will fall down after the injection. Practically, all induction combinations are based on one of two types of anaesthetic agent: a dissociative such as ketamine or tiletamine, or a barbiturate such as thiopental. Although the horse becomes unconscious after the induction agent is given, the course of induction is extremely dependent on the effects of premedication. In many cases, premedication forms part of the induction process.

The anaesthetic agent alters the way in which the horse becomes recumbent. Following thiopental injection the horse tends to go backwards, the head goes up, and, if not restrained, the animal may 'go over backwards'. However, it is usually easy to push the horse in the desired direction and, if in a recovery box, it will back into and slide down the wall. In contrast, following ketamine combinations all four legs of the horse may buckle and it will sink to the ground (see Figure 3.1). Although this usually leads to a very controlled induction, sometimes the horse will walk forward, and if this happens it is very difficult to control. A number of effective methods can be used to control the horse as it becomes recumbent (Chapter 7, pages 123–129), but the handler needs to be aware of the difference between the two types of induction drug in order to anticipate how the horse will fall.

ANAESTHETIC AGENTS AND COMBINATIONS USED FOR INDUCTION

KETAMINE

Ketamine is a so-called dissociative anaesthetic now widely used in equine anaesthesia. It is not suitable alone for induction of anaesthesia in horses as it may cause seizures. It is therefore essential to ensure that it is not accidentally given before the sedative. After suitable premedication it has

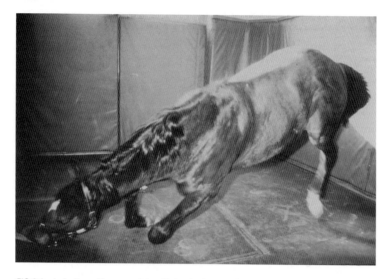

FIG 3.1 Induction with α₂ agonist and ketamine is generally smooth; the horse usually buckles at the knees before sitting back and going into sternal recumbency.

proved its worth for use in horses. Cardiovascular and respiratory depression are minimal and analgesia is good. After appropriate premedication, relaxation is good and recovery generally smooth, if sometimes abrupt. Solutions are not irritant to IV injection.

Ketamine anaesthesia is unusual in that the eyes remain open and central for some minutes after IV injection, making assessment of the depth of anaesthesia more difficult. It is metabolised by the liver and excreted by the kidney, and is less cumulative than thiopental. Incremental doses do not noticeably prolong recovery, although cumulation occurs. It is generally used after premedication with α_2 agonists, guaiphenesin, a benzodiazepine, or a combination of two or more of these. Some examples are given below.

α_2 Agonist and ketamine
Xylazine (1 mg/kg) or detomidine (0.01–0.02 mg/kg) or romifidine (0.1 mg/kg) and ketamine (2 mg/kg). This technique can be used with or without acepromazine premedication. The α_2 agonist is given IV and must be allowed to take full effect (5 minutes). Ketamine is then given as a single bolus injection and the horse is restrained quietly but firmly. It is essential that the

horse is not disturbed by noise or sudden movement at this stage, or induction may be violent. The horse should be kept with its head straight in front of the body and not allowed to move around. However, the handler should not push against the horse, as it will tend to push against the restraint and come forwards as it lies down. With firm but tactful restraint the horse should buckle at the knees and then sink back into sternal then lateral recumbency in a slow, controlled manner (Figure 3.1). Relaxation may be slow to develop and the horse should be allowed to settle for at least 30 seconds after it has gone into lateral recumbency (Figure 3.2). Anaesthesia can be maintained for

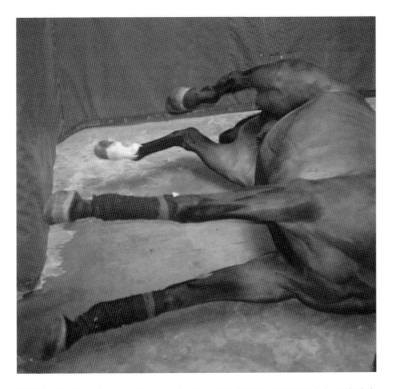

FIG 3.2 *After ketamine induction, once the horse has become recumbent it is particularly important that it is allowed to relax completely before it is handled or moved. The non-dependent limbs will slowly sink to the ground over the next 30–60 seconds. If the horse is handled too soon good relaxation may not develop at all, and it may even try to get up.*

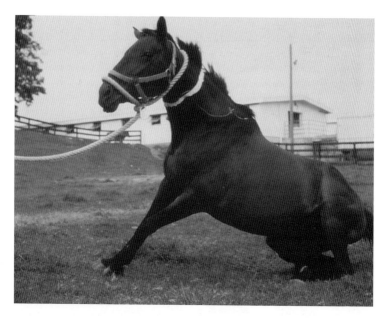

FIG 3.3 α₂-Agonist and ketamine anaesthesia usually leads to a quiet recovery if the horse is allowed to become fully relaxed after induction and is left to get up in its own time.

a short period with incremental doses of various induction agents, and such techniques are commonly used for minor procedures under 'field' conditions (pages 47–52). Recovery is generally smooth (Figure 3.3).

α₂ Agonist, ketamine and benzodiazepine

Xylazine (0.75–1 mg/kg) or detomidine (0.01–0.02 mg/kg) or romifidine (0.08–0.1 mg/kg) and diazepam (0.01–0.2 mg/kg) or midazolam (0.01–0.2 mg/kg) and ketamine 2 mg/kg. This technique has become popular, as without the benzodiazepine, anaesthesia and relaxation are sometimes inadequate and recovery abrupt. The addition of benzodiazepine appears to improve relaxation, particularly in a horse that was unsettled before induction, or in a disturbing environment. It must be remembered that benzodiazepines alone cause marked ataxia and muscle weakness, and the anaesthetic must be given immediately after the benzodiazepine. Ketamine and the benzodiazepine are often mixed, avoiding this problem. No undesirable effects of such mixtures have been reported, although technical data on drug compatibility are unknown. The lower doses of benzodiazepines are used with the higher doses of α_2 agonist (and vice versa). The technique can be used with or without acepromazine (0.03–0.05 mg/kg) premedication. The α_2 agonist is given and allowed to take effect (5 minutes). The benzodiazepine is given either immediately before, together with or immediately after the ketamine. The horse must be held still after the benzodiazepine/ketamine combination has been given as there may be a brief period of ataxia before it becomes unconscious. The horse normally sinks smoothly into sternal then lateral recumbency, and relaxation develops more quickly than when α_2 agonist/ ketamine is used alone. Anaesthesia can be maintained for short procedures with incremental doses of various induction agents described under 'field' conditions (pages 47–52).

Guaiphenesin and ketamine

Guaiphenesin (50–100 mg/kg) and ketamine (2 mg/kg). This is a suitable combination to be used when α_2 agonists are contraindicated. In healthy horses this technique is best used after acepromazine (0.03–0.05 mg/kg) premedication. In toxic horses the combination of guaiphenesin and ketamine is ideal. Guaiphenesin is infused rapidly until the horse becomes ataxic (Figure 3.4). The horse should be well restrained during infusion so that it does not panic when ataxia develops. The dose that can be given depends on the amount of support given to the horse. If the animal is well supported by handlers, a swinging door or a tilt table (pages 124–129), 75–100 mg/kg can be given before induction of anaesthesia. If the horse is less well supported up to 50 mg/kg is given. Ketamine is then injected as a bolus and the horse sinks into sternal and then lateral recumbency. This technique may not produce anaesthesia deep enough for minor procedures, although it is usually adequate for induction before transition to volatile agent maintenance.

With α_2 agonist: xylazine (0.5 mg/kg) or detomidine (0.01 mg/kg) or romifidine (0.05 mg/kg) and guaiphenesin (25–50 mg/kg) and ketamine (2 mg/kg). This can be used with or without acepromazine (0.03–0.05 mg/kg) premedication. The α_2 agonist is given IV and allowed to take effect, then guaiphenesin is infused as above and ketamine given as a bolus when the horse has become mildly ataxic. The α_2 agonist induces some ataxia so the dose of guaiphenesin is reduced, but it is more difficult to judge the degree

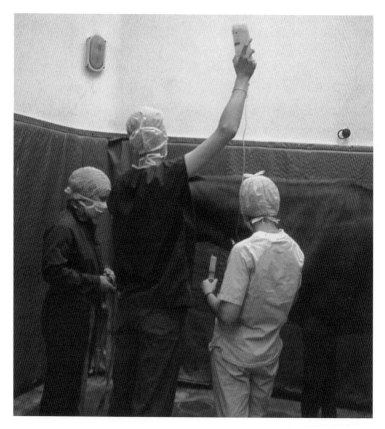

FIG 3.4   Guaiphenesin must be given by infusion.

of ataxia. This technique leads to smoother, more controlled induction of anaesthesia than using guaiphenesin/ketamine alone. Anaesthesia is best prolonged for short additional periods with further doses of ketamine (0.2 mg/kg) and guaiphenesin (5 mg/kg).

With benzodiazepine: guaiphenesin (25–50 mg/kg) and diazepam (0.05–0.1 mg/kg) or midazolam (0.05–0.1 mg/kg) and ketamine (2 mg/kg). This can be used with or without acepromazine (0.03–0.05 mg/kg) premedication. In restless horses it is best used with acepromazine so that the horse relaxes during the infusion. Guaiphenesin is infused until the horse is only slightly ataxic; lower doses are required than when only ketamine is used. The benzodiazepine is then given as a single slow bolus injection, either immediately before or from the same syringe as the ketamine. Induction is usually smooth and calm, but the horse must be prevented from walking immediately after the benzodiazepine/ketamine injection has been given or a brief period of ataxia and excitement may be seen. Anaesthesia is best prolonged for short additional periods with further doses of ketamine (0.2 mg/kg) and guaiphenesin (5 mg/kg).

With α_2 agonist, benzodiazepine and ketamine. Various combinations of all four drugs can be used together to induce anaesthesia. The doses of each are adjusted to produce the overall effect, but ketamine usually remains at 2 mg/kg. Commonly, the lower doses of the α_2 agonist (xylazine 0.5 mg/kg; detomidine 0.01 mg/kg; romifidine 0.05 mg/kg) and the benzodiazepines (diazepam 0.05 mg/kg or midazolam 0.05 mg/kg) are used. The α_2 agonist is given and allowed to take effect. Guaiphenesin (25–50 mg/kg) is then infused and the benzodiazepine is given immediately before or with ketamine (2 mg/kg). This drug combination is used routinely in some clinics, which find that the combined effect of all the drugs produces the most controlled induction. Prolongation for short periods is best carried out with additional ketamine (0.2 mg/kg) and guaiphenesin (5 mg/kg).

TILETAMINE

Tiletamine, a drug from the same group as ketamine, is commercially available (Zoletil, Telazol) in a number of countries in a fixed (50:50) combination with zolazepam, another benzodiazepine. The concept is similar to the combination of diazepam or midazolam with ketamine. It is generally used in combination with xylazine or detomidine and produces short-duration anaesthesia not dissimilar to, but with a more prolonged duration than that produced by the α_2-agonist–benzodiazepine–ketamine combinations described above. A number of different dose regimens have been advocated; the higher the doses the longer the duration of anaesthesia but the greater the chance of poor-quality recovery. Acepromazine (0.03–0.05 mg/kg) may be used as a premedicant and has been shown to improve subsequent cardiopulmonary function.

Xylazine (1.0 mg/kg) or detomidine (0.01–0.02 mg/kg) and tiletamine/ zolazepam (1.0–2.0 mg/kg total drug, i.e. 0.5–1.0 mg/kg of each agent). Xylazine or detomidine is given IV and the horse allowed to become fully sedated.

The tiletamine/zolazepam combination is then given as a bolus IV and anaesthesia is induced in a similar manner to that seen with the other α_2-agonist–benzodiazepine–ketamine combinations. The same firm but tactful restraint on the head is required. This produces 20–30 minutes of anaesthesia and generally a smooth recovery.

THIOPENTAL

Thiopental is a barbiturate that has been used in equine anaesthesia for many years. Without premedication, IV doses of 12–15 mg/kg rapidly induce anaesthesia. A single dose gives around 10 minutes' anaesthesia and may lead to an ataxic and excitable recovery, so it is more usual to use the agent at a reduced dosage following sedative premedication. Thiopental depresses respiration and blood pressure, but the effect is short-lived and of little consequence in a healthy horse. These effects are greatly enhanced in the presence of endotoxaemia. Solutions of thiopental are highly irritant and must not be given by perivascular injection; a catheter is advised. Solutions should be as dilute as the volume will allow. In many cases a 5% solution is practicable, but in large horses a 10% solution may be required.

Recovery from thiopental anaesthesia depends on recirculation of the drug from the brain into other tissues, but metabolism is slow. Incremental doses lead to a prolonged recovery. Thiopental is highly protein bound and the effective dose is reduced in foals and hypoproteinaemic horses. Thiopental does not have intrinsic analgesic properties and is now rarely used alone. It is better used after premedication, which, if heavy, allows a significant reduction of the induction dose.

Acepromazine and thiopental

Acepromazine (0.03–0.05 mg/kg) is given IV at least 15 minutes (or 45 min if IM) before thiopental (10–12 mg/kg). Thiopental is given as a single bolus injection. The horse tends to pull back, but with good control on the head it can be encouraged to go into sternal and then lateral recumbency.

Guaiphenesin and thiopental

This technique is best used after acepromazine (0.03–0.05 mg/kg) or low-dose α_2-agonist (xylazine 0.5 mg/kg, detomidine 0.01 mg/kg, romifidine 0.05 mg/kg) premedication. Guaiphenesin (25–100 mg) is infused rapidly until the horse becomes ataxic. The maximum dose depends on the amount of support given to the horse, with higher doses possible if more support is given.

Thiopental (5–6 mg/kg) is then injected as a bolus and the horse normally sinks quietly into sternal and then lateral recumbency. Induction of anaesthesia may also be carried out with 2.5 g thiopental added to a bottle of 10% guaiphenesin, and this is infused until the horse goes down. This combination makes it more difficult to judge when the horse will go down and the procedure tends to be less well controlled in inexperienced hands. Anaesthesia can be maintained for a short period with incremental doses of guaiphenesin and thiopental. It is preferable that the total dose does not exceed 100 mg/kg guaiphenesin and 10 mg/kg thiopental, or the horse's recovery will be prolonged and ataxic.

α_2 *Agonist and thiopental*

Xylazine 1 mg/kg or detomidine 0.02 mg/kg or romifidine 0.1 mg/kg and thiopental 5–6 mg/kg. This technique can be used with or without acepromazine (0.03–0.05 mg/kg) premedication. The α_2 agonist is given IV and allowed to take effect (5 minutes). Thiopental is given as a slow single injection and the horse restrained firmly until it becomes recumbent. This takes considerably longer (1–2 min) than after acepromazine only, and the horse may paddle the legs gently before relaxing. Anaesthesia can be prolonged with incremental doses of thiopental, but the total dose should not exceed 11 mg/kg. Induction of anaesthesia with lower doses of the α_2 agonist (approximately half that recommended above) followed by 7–8 mg/kg thiopental also works well, being faster and slightly more predictable.

TOTAL INTRAVENOUS ANAESTHESIA (TIVA)

Total intravenous anaesthesia is widely used in medicine for major surgery. In horses such techniques are in their infancy, but they have considerable attraction for this species as volatile agents cause so much cardiovascular and respiratory depression. In general, cardiovascular depression, particularly as manifest by hypotension, is less marked with intravenous anaesthesia. However, respiratory depression may still occur and oxygen supplementation should still be available. The major problem with TIVA is that many of the agents used are cumulative, so that after prolonged anaesthesia recovery can be slow and of poor quality.

'TRIPLE DRIP'

The TIVA technique most commonly used at present is the so-called 'triple drip'. This is a combination of an α_2 agonist, usually xylazine or detomidine, with guaiphenesin and ketamine. Although all three drugs are relatively cumulative (particularly guaiphenesin) the technique has proved extremely useful for maintenance of anaesthesia in horses. It is most commonly used to prolong field anaesthesia in a controlled manner (Figure 3.5), but it has also been used for major surgery. It is probably better restricted to procedures lasting less than 2 hours, as beyond this guaiphenesin accumulates, leading to an ataxic recovery. Cardiovascular and respiratory depression are minimal, surgical conditions are good and recovery is usually smooth. Recovery may be

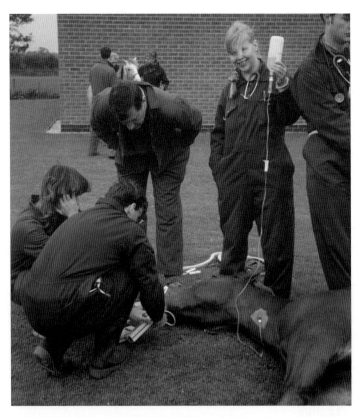

FIG 3.5 *"Triple drip", a combination of guaiphenesin, ketamine and an α_2 agonist, can be used to maintain anaesthesia in a controlled manner without volatile agents. In this case it is used to maintain anaesthesia for castration.*

slightly longer than after halothane and is sometimes ataxic, but excitement is rare. The α_2 agonist component blocks insulin release and causes hyperglycaemia and diuresis. Copious volumes of urine are produced.

Technique

The best-documented solution contains guaiphenesin 100 mg/mL, detomidine 0.02 mg/mL (or xylazine 1 mg/mL) and ketamine 2 mg/mL. This is made up by adding 1 g ketamine and 10 mg detomidine (500 mg xylazine) to 500 mL of 10% guaiphenesin. However, solutions containing less guaiphenesin at 50 mg/mL have proved very satisfactory, and are less irritant and less cumulative. This solution is made up by using 5% instead of 10% guaiphenesin. Anaesthesia is induced by any standard method, but preferably one that does not incorporate guaiphenesin so that the total dose of this drug is kept as low as possible. Anaesthesia is maintained by an infusion of approximately 1 mL/kg/h of the solution. Higher rates may be needed for the first 10–15 minutes and the rate should be almost halved after 60 minutes. The infusion is stopped in the same way as halothane administration is stopped when surgery has been completed. For procedures longer than 20–30 minutes the horse should be intubated and allowed to breathe oxygen. Respiratory rate is well maintained and oxygen-enriched air is sufficient. This can be provided by insufflating oxygen into the distal end of the endotracheal tube at 10–15 L/min.

CLIMAZOLAM–KETAMINE ANAESTHESIA

A technique using an infusion of climazolam, a long-acting benzodiazepine, in combination with ketamine has been used successfully for maintenance of anaesthesia in Switzerland, where climazolam is available. This combination causes even less cardiovascular and respiratory depression than the triple drip and has been widely used for a range of major surgery lasting up to 2 hours. Climazolam is long acting and its effect is reversed with the benzodiazepine antagonist sarmazenil, also available in Switzerland. Recovery is normally very smooth, although occasionally horses may appear slightly disorientated.

Technique

This is generally used after induction of anaesthesia with xylazine (1 mg/kg) and ketamine (2.0 mg/kg IV). Climazolam (0.2 mg/kg) is given IV 2 minutes after the ketamine injection. Anaesthesia is then maintained with an infusion of climazolam 0.4 mg/kg/h and ketamine 6.0 mg/kg/h. The infusion is stopped when surgery ends. In order to let the effects of ketamine abate before the benzodiazepine antagonist is given, sarmazenil (0.04 mg/kg) is given IV 20 minutes after the infusion is stopped. Recovery then occurs within a few minutes. Oxygen should be given but can be insufflated into the endotracheal tube.

PROPOFOL ANAESTHESIA

Propofol is a non-cumulative intravenous anaesthetic, widely used in humans and small animals, which has many attributes that make it highly suitable for total intravenous anaesthesia in horses. At present, cost prevents routine clinical use, but combinations with α_2 agonists and/or ketamine have proved satisfactory.

Propofol/medetomidine

This technique has been used very satisfactorily under both experimental and clinical conditions to maintain anaesthesia for periods of up to 4 hours. Medetomidine is off label but short acting and non-cumulative in the horse, and is chosen primarily for its excellent analgesic properties. Induction of anaesthesia is with medetomidine (7 μg/kg) followed by ketamine (2.2 mg/kg); maintenance uses a continuous-rate infusion of 3.5 μg/kg/min medetomidine, and propofol to effect (starting at 0.1 mg/kg/min). There is little cardiovascular depression, but respiratory depression means that oxygen insufflation is required. It takes practice to judge the depth of anaesthesia with this combination: horses appear very lightly anaesthestised and may blink and have nystagmus, yet do not respond to surgery. A further 2 μg/kg medetomidine is given for recovery, which is generally rapid and of good quality; there is no need to reverse the medetomidine. As with all techniques infusing α_2 agonists, copious urine is produced.

Propofol–xylazine infusions have been used experimentally but doses suitable for clinical use have not yet been fully elucidated.

Propofol/ketamine

Ketamine has been infused with propofol to maintain anaesthesia in horses. This provides stable anaesthesia with good cardiovascular function, but respiratory depression may still be a problem. A loading dose of propofol (0.3 mg/kg) is given, followed by infusion at 0.16 mg/kg/min. The infusion rate is reduced by 0.01 mg/kg/min after 60 minutes, and then every 30 minutes until it is given at 0.1 mg/kg/min. Ketamine is infused at 0.04 mg/kg/min for 60 minutes and then progressively reduced by 0.01 mg/kg/min every 30–40 minutes until 0.02 mg/kg/min is reached. Ketamine infusion should be stopped 30 minutes before the end of surgery. Recovery is generally smooth, but marked nystagmus may be seen during the first 5–10 minutes and the horse must not be allowed to attempt to stand until this ceases.

FIELD ANAESTHESIA

An ideal field anaesthetic provides short, good-quality anaesthesia followed by a rapid recovery and return to normality, so the horse can safely be left in the care of its owner. Although no ideal field anaesthetic exists, many of the intravenous induction techniques described above are successfully used alone for anaesthesia 'in the field' for short procedures such as castration. Although the surgery is minor and may last only a few minutes, general anaesthesia is employed and the horse must be adequately monitored.

The aim is to ensure that the ABC is cared for: **A**irway, **B**reathing and **C**irculation. Sophisticated monitoring is not required, but respiration must be observed so that obstruction or apnoea is noticed before it is too late. The pulse should be palpated regularly. Small portable pulse oximeters are a useful but not essential non-invasive monitor to use under field conditions (Figure 3.6).

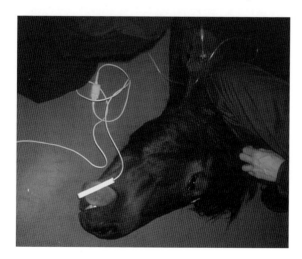

FIG 3.6 A portable pulse oximeter is a valuable aid to monitoring field anaesthesia when the pony is breathing air. If oxygenation is adequate this indicates that respiration is adequate. The oximeter also monitors the quality of the peripheral pulse.

In a horse breathing air, pulse oximetry provides relevant information about both respiration and the state of the peripheral circulation.

An IV catheter should be placed. This may be necessary for administration of irritant solutions, but it is also there to allow further administration of anaesthetic drugs if anaesthesia becomes too light, and for emergency use if disaster occurs.

Ideally, whenever any animal is given a general anaesthetic some means of resuscitation should be readily available, particularly to treat apnoea. It is a relatively simple matter to take an endotracheal tube and a small oxygen cylinder (size E) with a demand valve (Figure 3.7). Even a large horse can be ventilated by this means for 10–20 minutes. This is long enough to keep the horse ventilated until spontaneous respiration returns after apnoea was induced by an IV anaesthetic. A portable to-and-fro circuit can also be used for manual ventilation.

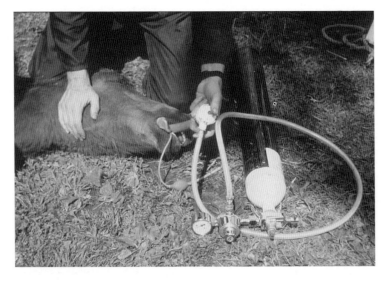

FIG 3.7   A demand valve attached to a small oxygen cylinder is a portable system for supplying oxygen, for support of ventilation and for resuscitation. The demand valve is triggered by the horse's own respiration or can be controlled manually, as illustrated.

A suitable site for field anaesthesia must be chosen. In good weather a well-covered flat grass field or lawn is ideal (Figure 3.8). Bricks and other hazards should be removed. Alternatively, an all-weather indoor or outdoor arena may be used. This provides good grip for the horse but dusty conditions for surgery. Most horses can also safely be anaesthetised in a large strong loosebox with smooth walls and deep bedding.

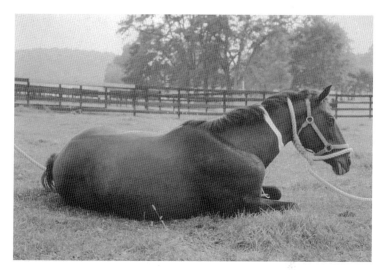

FIG 3.8   *A safe site must be used for field anaesthesia. In good weather a flat field is suitable.*

KETAMINE AND BARBITURATE TECHNIQUES

The techniques used in the field are generally based on either ketamine or thiopental anaesthesia, preceded by α_2-agonist or guaiphenesin premedication. Benzodiazepines may also be included. The techniques are described above and those most suitable for field use are summarised in Table 3.1.

All the techniques described can be preceded by acepromazine premedication (0.03 mg/kg), with or without butophanol if desired. This is a useful approach in nervous, highly strung animals and undoubtedly smoothes the whole procedure. In this case the acepromazine should be given IV at least 15 minutes (30–40 min if IM) before induction of anaesthesia, before surgical equipment is made ready.

Table 3.1 Recommended techniques for field anaesthesia

Ketamine-based anaesthesia – premedication with α₂ agonists

α₂	α₂ dose	Ketamine dose	Duration of anaesthesia	Prolongation	Comment
Xylazine	1 mg/kg	2 mg/kg	10–20 min	Thio 1–2 mg/kg Xyl+ ket: half induction dose 'Triple drip'* 1 mL/kg/min	Slow induction Good resp Good cardiovasc Relaxation usually good but variable Recovery smooth but abrupt
Detomidine	0.015–0.02 mg/kg	2 mg/kg	10–25 min	Thio 1–2 mg/kg Ket 0.5–1 mg 'Triple drip'* 1 mL/kg/min	Slow induction Good resp Good cardiovasc Relaxation usually good but variable Recovery smooth but abrupt
Romifidine	0.08–0.1 mg/kg	2 mg/kg	10–25 min	Thio 1–2 mg/kg Ket 0.5–1 mg 'Triple drip'* 1 mL/kg/min	Slow induction Good resp Good cardiovasc Relaxation usually good but variable Recovery smooth but abrupt

Variations: use of benzodiazepines

Any α_2 as above	Dose as above	Give diazepam 0.01–0.05 mg at same time as ket 2 mg/kg	Additional 5–10 min	As above	Slow induction Occasional apnoea at induc Good cardiovasc Relaxation good Recovery smooth, less abrupt

Variations: use of butorphanol

Any of α_2 as above	Dose as above	Give butorph 0.02 mg/kg at same time as α_2	Additional 5–10 min	As above	Slow induction Good resp but watch carefully Good cardiovasc Relaxation good Recovery smooth

Continued

Table 3.1 Recommended techniques for field anaesthesia—cont'd

Thiopental-based anesthesia – premedication with α_2 agonists

α_2	α_2 dose	Thiopent dose	Duration of anaesthesia	Prolongation	Comment
Xylazine	1 mg/kg	5 mg/kg	15–20 min	Thio 1–2 mg/kg 'Triple drip'* 1 mL/kg/min	Slow induction Good resp Good cardiovasc Relaxation usually good Recovery smooth
Detomidine	0.015–0.02 mg/kg	5 mg/kg	15–25 min	Thio 1–2 mg/kg 'Triple drip'* 1 mL/kg/min	Slow induction Good resp Good cardiovasc Relaxation usually good Recovery smooth
Romifidine	0.08–0.1 mg/kg	5 mg/kg	15–25 min	Thio 1–2 mg/kg 'Triple drip'* 1 mL/kg/min	Slow induction Good resp Good cardiovasc Relaxation usually good Recovery smooth

Thiopental-based anaesthesia – premedication with guaiphenesin

	Guaiph.	Thiopent dose	Duration of anaesthesia	Prolongation	Comment
Guaiphenesin	25–75 mg/kg by infusion	5 mg/kg	15–20 min	Thio 1–2 mg/kg Thio 1–2 mg/kg and guaiph 5 mg/kg 'Triple drip'*	Best preceded by aceprom premed: more control at induction Induction after thio 30 s Good resp Good cardiovasc Relaxation usually good Recovery may be ataxic

Variations: premedication with α_2 *agonists*

	Guaiph.	Thiopent dose	Duration of anaesthesia	Prolongation	Comment
Premed with α_2 agent: xyl 0.5 mg/kg det 0.01mg/kg rom 0.05mg/kg	As above guaiph 25–50 mg/kg by infusion	As above	20–30 min	As above	As above but more control at induction, though may be more ataxic

*Triple drip: 500 mL guaiphenesin 5 or 10% + 1 g ketamine + 10 mg detomidine, or 500 mL guaiphenesin + 1 g ketamine + 500 mg xylazine. NB. Some commercial solutions of guaiphenesin are 15%. Appropriate adjustments should be made so that the same drug doses are given. The quality and duration of anaesthesia in all cases is improved by the additional use of appropriate local anaesthetic techniques.

The 'triple drip' is a valuable addition to field anaesthesia and can be used to prolong anaesthesia in a controlled manner when the induction technique alone provides insufficient time (see Figure 3.5).

OTHER METHODS FOR FIELD ANAESTHESIA

Immobilon is the trade name for a combination of etorphine, an extremely potent opioid (2.45 mg/mL), and acepromazine (10 mg/mL) marketed for anaesthesia in horses and large exotics. In horses it produces a particular type of anaesthesia where analgesia is good, relaxation is poor, respiration is severely depressed and the cardiovascular system works overtime owing to tachycardia and spectacular hypertension. The horse's eyes remain open and the lower one must be protected against abrasion from the surface on which the horse is lying. Sweating may be profuse, making conditions unsuitable for clipping. Priapism occurs occasionally (Figure 3.9) and care must be taken to

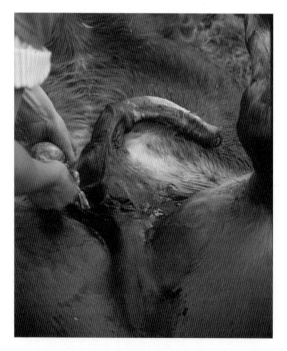

FIG 3.9   Immobilon may cause penile engorgement and priapism, as shown here during castration.

ensure the penis is not damaged. The main advantage of Immobilon anaesthesia is that the etorphine is reversed by the opioid antagonist diprenorphine, which is given at the end of surgery. Etorphine is rapidly fatal if injected into humans and requires extreme care in handling. Naloxone, the pure opioid antagonist, should always be readily available when Immobilon is used, and a second person must be instructed in its use in case of inadvertent injection of the veterinary surgeon.

Chloral hydrate used to be widely used in equine anaesthesia but became less popular because of its irritancy and the large volume required. However, if given through a catheter (to ensure that it does not go subcutaneously) it could still be regarded as having a place in equine anaesthesia. Chloral hydrate (as a 10% or less solution) is infused until the horse becomes ataxic (25–50 mg/kg). Thiopental (5 mg/kg) or ketamine (2 mg/kg) is then given IV to induce anaesthesia. Local analgesia should be used appropriate to the surgery. Recovery may be ataxic, particularly if anaesthesia was prolonged.

Further reading

Baker KL, Taylor PM, Fowden AL and Bloomfield M (1999) Propofol-ketamine anaesthesia in late gestation ponies. *Journal of Veterinary Anaesthesia* **26**: 45.

Bettschart-Wolfensberger R, Kalchofner K, Neges K, et al (2005) Total intravenous anaesthesia in horses using medetomidine and propofol. *Veterinary Anaesthesia and Analgesia* **32**: 348–354.

Bettschart-Wolfensberger R, Taylor PM, Sear JW, et al (1996) Physiologic effects of anesthesia induced and maintained by intravenous administration of a climazolam-ketamine combination in ponies premedicated with acepromazine and xylazine. *American Journal of Veterinary Research* **57**: 1472–1477.

Hall LW, Clarke KW and Trim CM (2001) *Veterinary Anaesthesia*, 10th edn. WB Saunders, London.

Thurmon JC, Tranquilli WJ and Benson GJ (1996) *Lumb and Jones' Veterinary Anaesthesia*, 3rd edn. Williams & Wilkins, Baltimore, 210–240, 241–296.

Muir WW and Hubbell JAE (1991). *Muir and Hubbell's Equine Anaesthesia: Monitoring and Emergency Therapy.* Mosby Year Book, St Louis, 281–309.

Taylor PM, Kirby JJ, Shrimpton DJ, et al (1998) Cardiovascular effects of surgical castration during anesthesia maintained with halothane or infusion of detomidine, ketamine and guaiphenesin in ponies. *Equine Veterinary Journal* **30**: 304–309.

4

INHALATION ANAESTHESIA

In horses, anaesthesia for prolonged procedures is usually maintained by inhalation of a volatile anaesthetic agent. The drugs are potent and must be used with care. However, the easy control of administration, no defined limit to the duration of use and predictable recovery characteristics have made them indispensable in equine anaesthesia.

PHARMACOLOGY OF INHALATION ANAESTHETICS

UPTAKE AND ELIMINATION

Inhaled anaesthetics are absorbed into the blood through the pulmonary circulation and taken to the brain, where they cause anaesthesia. The depth of anaesthesia is proportional to the tension or pressure they exert in the brain, not to the mass of the drug in the body. During administration, the tension of a very soluble drug in the brain takes a long time to rise, as large quantities are absorbed by other tissues in the body. The tension of a less soluble drug rises much faster, as it has nowhere else to go. Thus a less soluble drug induces anaesthesia faster than a soluble drug. This counterintuitive feature of inhalation anaesthesia has important practical implications as it affects the speed of induction and recovery. Induction also can be hastened by anything that increases the rate of rise of the anaesthetic tension in the blood leaving the lungs. Hence higher inspired concentrations and increased respiration speed up induction, although doing so rapidly may cause unacceptable cardiovascular depression. Recovery is similar, but in reverse. However, because the inspired concentration cannot be taken below zero, the effect of a high diffusion gradient cannot be used to remove the drug from the body in the way that a high inspired concentration is used to increase the gradient during induction. Inhalation anaesthetics are redistributed into fat, and for agents with high fat solubility this will delay recovery, the effect being clinically noticeable particularly after long-duration anaesthesia.

MINIMUM ALVEOLAR CONCENTRATION (MAC)

The MAC of any anaesthetic is the concentration (at atmospheric pressure) that prevents 50% of animals moving in response to a supramaximal noxious stimulus. MAC is thus a measure of the potency of the inhalation anaesthetic agents; it is used to compare the potency of different drugs and, more importantly, to compare side effects at equipotent doses. Since the depth of anaesthesia is related to brain tension and brain tension is proportional to alveolar concentration, the alveolar concentration (taken as end-tidal concentration and practicable to monitor) is used as a measure of the depth of anaesthesia. Standards texts state that when an inhalation agent is used alone, approximately 1.5 MAC is needed for surgery. This appears true for halothane, but with the newer agents, lower MAC multiples seem to be adequate. In practice, the inhalation agents are rarely used alone; concurrent use of sedatives, injectable anaesthetic and analgesic agents, as well as analgesia using local anaesthetic blocks reduce the required dose.

THE ANAESTHETIC AGENTS

ISOFLURANE

Isoflurane is now the most widely used inhalation agent for equine anaesthesia, and holds a marketing authorisation for this purpose in both North America and Europe. Isoflurane is non-flammable, easily vaporised, and has both lower blood and lower fat solubility than the previously used agent, halothane. The physical properties enable rapid induction and stabilisation of anaesthesia, but also mean it is easy to overdose. The MAC of isoflurane is close to 1.2%, and following premedication and intravenous induction an alveolar (thus end-tidal) concentration of 1.3–1.5% is usually sufficient to maintain anaesthesia for surgery. Recovery from anaesthetics of short or moderate duration is rapid (15–20 minutes), but the fat solubility is such that after prolonged anaesthesia (4 hours or more) recovery is noticeably slower. Recovery from isoflurane anaesthesia is sometimes associated with disorientation and a degree of violence, so it is common to reduce the risk of this by the judicious use of sedation (pages 161–163).

Isoflurane affects most other body systems, the most significant being the cardiovascular and respiratory systems. It causes peripheral vasodilation and hence hypotension, which can be severe. At alveolar levels close to MAC there is little myocardial depression, so peripheral blood flow is good, as indicated by the appearance of pink mucous membranes. Myocardial depression does occur at higher doses. Isoflurane does not sensitise the heart to catecholamine-induced dysrhythmias.

Isoflurane is a potent respiratory depressant. Tidal volume is often high, but the respiratory rate very low. The respiratory centre is depressed, the response to rising carbon dioxide reduced, and hypoxia becomes the major respiratory drive. The respiratory depression is often such as to slow the uptake of isoflurane, and it can be difficult to obtain adequate anaesthesia without the use of intermittent positive-pressure ventilation (IPPV) (pages 76–77).

Metabolism
Very little isoflurane is metabolised in the liver, most being exhaled unchanged. This makes isoflurane relatively safe for the anaesthetist, who inevitably occasionally inspires some of the drug. Any benefit to the horse from this feature is hypothetical.

HALOTHANE
Halothane, first used in equine anaesthesia in 1957, enabled the achievement of prolonged anaesthesia followed by a smooth, predictable recovery. Without such anaesthesia, equine surgery would not have developed to its current degree of sophistication. Halothane is now rarely used in human anaesthesia and is no longer available in the USA. However, epidemiological studies have demonstrated that for equine anaesthesia the overall safety of halothane and that of isoflurane are equal. Halothane's main disadvantage in horses is the degree of myocardial depression produced. Its advantages are the ability to maintain spontaneous respiration, and that in most cases its use is followed by a smooth and quiet recovery.

Halothane is a potent anaesthetic that is not irritant to the respiratory tract. It is non-flammable, but is light sensitive and stored in dark bottles with thymol as preservative. It is more soluble in both blood and fat than is isoflurane, so induction and recovery are a little slower, although induction can be speeded up by the use of high inspired concentrations. The MAC of halothane is close to 0.8%. This means that an alveolar (end-tidal; see pages 55–56) concentration of 0.8–1.2% should be sufficient to maintain anaesthesia for surgery after most common induction techniques. Recovery from halothane anaesthesia is usually smooth and calm, and the use of additional sedation is not necessarily required.

Halothane affects most other body systems, the most significant being the cardiovascular and respiratory systems. It is a potent myocardial depressant, leading to dose-dependent decreases in cardiac output and hypotension. It causes little vasodilation, so the decreased cardiac output causes hypotension. Halothane sensitises the heart to catecholamine-induced dysrhythmias. Halothane, like all inhalation anaesthetic agents, causes respiratory depression by reducing the response to carbon dioxide, whereas the response to hypoxia is usually unimpaired. Both tidal volume and respiratory rate decrease. However, respiratory depression is less than that of isoflurane and it is practicable to allow the horse to breathe spontaneously.

Metabolism

Although recovery from anaesthesia depends on exhalation of the drug, a certain amount is metabolised in the liver. The metabolites are responsible for some of the harmful effects of halothane in humans, although similar effects have not been reported in horses.

SEVOFLURANE

Sevoflurane is currently licensed in the USA and Europe for veterinary use in dogs, but not in horses. Nevertheless, there is now considerable experience of its use in this species. It is a potent volatile agent (MAC is approximately 2.8%) and is non-irritant to inhale. End-tidal concentrations of 2.8–3.0% are usually adequate to maintain stable anaesthesia. It has a lower blood and fat solubility than isoflurane, so induction and recovery from anaesthesia are very rapid, and it is easy to maintain a stable depth of anaesthesia. For those anaesthetists used to halothane and isoflurane, the rapid uptake of sevoflurane means that it is easy to overdose; high inspired concentrations should not be used to speed up induction if this is to be avoided. Recovery is fast, and, although believed calmer than after isoflurane, the rapidity may lead to disorientation and the horse may become violent. Judicious use of sedation (pages 161–163) will reduce or prevent poor-quality recoveries.

The cardiovascular and respiratory effects of sevoflurane are similar to those of isoflurane. Hypotension, which is dose-dependent, results from vasodilation, and cardiac function is well maintained. Experimental studies have demonstrated marked sevoflurane-induced cardiac depression with subsequent morbidity in individual animals, but such cases have not been reported from clinical trials. Sevoflurane does not sensitise the heart to catecholamine-induced dysrhythmias.

Metabolism and reactions with carbon dioxide absorbents

Hepatic metabolism and reactions with the classic carbon dioxide absorbents baralyme (now withdrawn) or soda lime mean there is a potential for renal toxicity. Extensive use in humans has not revealed any clinical problems, but new absorbents have been developed with which sevoflurane does not react.

DESFLURANE

Desflurane, a new volatile anaesthetic agent with solubility characteristics similar to those of nitrous oxide, is currently licensed for use in humans. Its low boiling point means it needs a special vaporiser. In horses, MAC is approximately 8%. Clinical experience suggests that, following intravenous induction of anaesthesia, end-tidal concentrations of between 7 and 9% are usually adequate to maintain stable anaesthesia. Induction is extremely fast and it is easy to maintain a constant depth of anaesthesia. To an even greater degree than sevoflurane it is also very easy to overdose, and there is no need to use high MAC multiples to speed up the transition from intravenous induction agents to inhalation anaesthesia. Clinical experience has shown that in the early stages of anaesthesia a vaporiser setting of 8–9% is sufficient. Recovery is very fast, as well as complete and calm; in clinical reports to date sedation has always been used, as this rapidity may lead to disorientation.

The cardiovascular effects of desflurane are similar to those of isoflurane. Hypotension, which is dose-dependent, results from vasodilation and cardiac function is well maintained. Desflurane does not sensitise the heart to catecholamine-induced dysrhythmias. Although desflurane causes dose-dependent respiratory depression, the degree appears less than that of isoflurane; it is usually practicable for the horse to breathe spontaneously.

Metabolism and reactions with carbon dioxide absorbents

Desflurane undergoes minimal metabolism in the body. In humans, when it is used with dry soda lime, carbon monoxide may accumulate in the anaesthetic circuit, but as so much moisture accumulates in equine anaesthetic circuits such breakdown products are unlikely to occur.

NITROUS OXIDE

Nitrous oxide is a gas at room temperature and is stored under pressure in cylinders, where it liquefies. It is one of the least soluble anaesthetic agents, so its maximum effect is rapidly achieved; elimination from the body is also rapid. It is not a potent drug (MAC is greater than 100%) but can be used to supplement the effects of the other volatile agents, in particular contributing excellent analgesic effects. Nitrous oxide's lack of potency means that high inspired concentrations are required to produce any effect, and that it therefore takes up a high proportion of the inspired gases, significantly (and potentially dangerously) reducing the inspired oxygen concentration. Nitrous oxide diffuses rapidly into gas-filled spaces in the body as it replaces nitrogen and thus increases the size of gas pockets. In horses this leads to abdominal distension, increased pressure on the lungs and increased ventilation/perfusion mismatch. On recovery, the rapid transfer of nitrous oxide from blood to alveolae reduces alveolar oxygen concentrations and may result in 'diffusion hypoxia'. As a consequence of all three of these factors, nitrous oxide is not universally used in horses.

Nitrous oxide is not irritant to the respiratory tract. In clinical use it has little cardiodepressant effect and does not sensitise the heart to catecholamine-induced dysrhythmias. It does not cause respiratory depression, but may lead to hypoxaemia as described above.

Nitrous oxide is a potent analgesic at subanaesthetic doses. Its value as a supplement to volatile-agent anaesthesia is probably a result of this attribute.

Nitrous oxide depresses bone marrow function, but this effect is only seen after several hours' administration and is not of clinical significance in horses. However, with prolonged exposure to low concentrations it has been shown to be teratogenic.

ANAESTHETIC EQUIPMENT

General anaesthesia always induces respiratory depression and a degree of hypoxaemia. Whether inhaled or intravenous anaesthesia is used, oxygen must be supplied for all but very short procedures. When volatile agents are used, complex equipment designed to vaporise the anaesthetic and to supply it to the lungs is essential. It is common practice to induce anaesthesia with IV agents and intubate the trachea while the horse is still anaesthetised with the IV agent. For maintenance of anaesthesia the tracheal tube is connected to a breathing circuit through which the anaesthetic agent is administered, vaporised in oxygen.

ENDOTRACHEAL INTUBATION

Horses are easy to intubate and tolerate the procedure well. Intubation goes a long way to ensuring a clear airway and is much easier to manage than a mask.

Cuffed endotracheal tube

These tubes have a cuff at the distal end which is inflated to produce an airtight seal between the tube and the trachea. They are inserted through the larynx into the trachea and should reach the mid to lower third of the cervical trachea (Figure 4.1). These tubes are made of silicone, red rubber or polythene. The silicone tube is probably the easiest to use and also to repair. Polythene tubes have a 'low-pressure' cuff, which may protect the tracheal lining but also makes them more difficult to introduce. The old red rubber tubes are robust but may cause more damage to the tracheal lining.

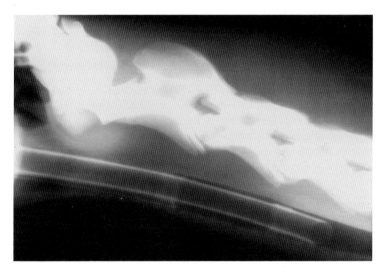

FIG 4.1   Radiograph of an anaesthetised horse with endotracheal tube in place. The distal end of the tube should reach the mid to lower third of the cervical trachea.

Insertion. Horses have a poor laryngeal reflex and the endotracheal tube (ETT) is passed through the mouth and larynx and into the trachea with minimal resistance. This is greatly facilitated if the head and neck are extended (Figure 4.2). Under normal circumstances the horse is a nose breather, so the

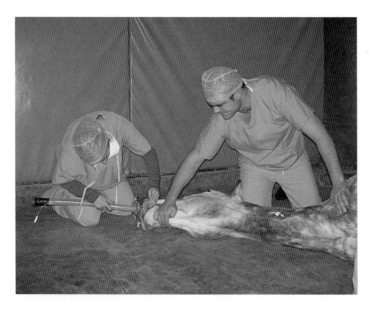

FIG 4.2 Intubation of the trachea. The horse is an obligate nose breather and under normal circumstances the tip of the epiglottis lies above the soft palate. With red rubber tubes, introduction of the endotracheal tube with the concave curve pointing dorsally helps to dislocate the soft palate from the epiglottis before the tube is turned through 90° and advanced on down the trachea with the concave curve ventrally. As seen here, with the straight silicone tubes now available simply extending the head is usually sufficient.

soft palate must be displaced dorsal to the epiglottis. With highly curved red rubber tubes this is most easily accomplished by passing the tube with the concave surface dorsally until it reaches the pharynx; the horse is heard to mouth breathe when the soft palate is displaced; the tube is then turned concave edge ventrally and passed smoothly into the trachea. The almost straight silicone tubes are more easily passed with any concavity positioned ventrally, at least until past the narrow space between the molar teeth. If the tube does not move easily it is either too large or in the wrong place, usually under the epiglottis. The position of the tip of the tube is readjusted by slight withdrawal to clear the epiglottis, further twisting, and another attempt is made. Positioning is often easiest if the tube can be advanced as the horse takes a breath. On no account should the tube be pushed forcibly or the pharynx, oesophagus or larynx may be damaged. When the tube enters the trachea it moves easily; if it has entered the oesophagus there is more resistance to its movement and the horse can be heard to mouth breathe. Differentiation between oesophageal and tracheal intubation is usually straightforward in horses: it is easy to detect gas breathed out of the tube when the horse expires. If necessary, the tube can be joined immediately to the breathing circuit and a couple of inspirations given manually. The chest wall rather than the abdomen should expand easily. This is better than compressing the chest and testing for expired gas coming down the tube. Once the tube is in place the breathing circuit is connected and the cuff inflated. Inflation should be just sufficient to prevent a gas leak around the tube when the rebreathing bag on the circuit is squeezed with the 'pop-off' spill valve closed. Higher cuff inflation pressures are not necessary and may damage the tracheal lining.

Size. The size of tube required is intuitively obvious from the size of the horse. Large Shires require 35 or even 40 mm, large hunters and warmbloods usually 30 mm, and 25–30 mm tubes are generally needed for full-grown Thoroughbreds; 20–24 mm tubes are better suited to young Thoroughbreds, ponies and cobs. Small ponies usually require 18–20 mm tubes. In Thoroughbred and horse breed foals, endotracheal tubes between 12 and 16 mm are required; smaller tubes may be needed for pony foals. The tubes used for foals need to be designed for the purpose: similar-diameter tubes supplied for large dogs are too short.

Cole tube

These are cuffless tubes with a stepped and tapered end, which is passed into the larynx. The step provides an airtight seal where it contacts the larynx. Although these tubes have the advantage of no cuff to maintain, they are more difficult to place accurately, are more likely to allow a leak around the tube, and may cause laryngeal damage.

Nasal tube

It is feasible to intubate the trachea via the nasal passages using a cuffed endotracheal tube. This procedure is commonly used in foals as the nasal passages are relatively large. It is also useful in adult horses to allow access to the mouth. A relatively smaller ETT is used and is passed blind in a similar manner to oral intubation.

BREATHING CIRCUIT

Breathing circuits used in equine anaesthesia are almost exclusively of the rebreathing type, where an absorbent (classically soda lime) is used to extract the exhaled carbon dioxide from the circuit before the gases are returned to the animal for the next inspiration. Non-rebreathing systems, where a high fresh gas flow pushes the expired carbon dioxide out of the system before the next breath, may occasionally be used in small foals. However, the size of most horses generally precludes the use of systems dependent on high fresh gas flows.

Soda lime absorbs carbon dioxide by an exothermic chemical reaction. The soda lime should become noticeably warm during the course of anaesthesia. In hot weather and with low-flow methods excess heat can be a problem, and it may be necessary to change the absorbent. Soda lime is an irritant compound and dust particles from the canister should be regularly cleaned out of the circuit to prevent them entering the horse's airway. Soda lime is also used up; it must be replaced when it is exhausted. It is commercially available with a dye indicator that causes the granules to change colour when they are exhausted. Two forms are commonly available and it is essential to know which is currently in use. One variety is coloured pink and goes white when used; the other is white and goes lilac when used. On no account should these be mixed, as it would severely confuse interpretation of the colour change. Soda lime is best used in transparent canisters so that the colour change is readily apparent. Used granules should be discarded immediately after use as the colour tends to revert when they are left standing, but the granules are still exhausted. Dye colour is also lost when the granules are wet.

Recently a number of new absorbents have been developed to reduce or negate the problem of toxic compounds being formed through reaction between anaesthetic agents and basic soda lime. These absorbents are considerably less dusty than the classic soda lime. The dye colours used to show exhaustion may differ from those described above. If sevoflurane is used in a low-flow system the use of one of these new absorbents is strongly recommended.

Two fundamental designs of rebreathing system are used: the to-and-fro and the circle system. Purpose-built large-animal systems with 5 cm diameter tubing are required for adult horses, but small-animal circles designed for use in adult humans are adequate for young foals. The absorbent is most efficiently used if it is packed in a canister where the gases flow vertically; this prevents the gases from tracking along a granule-free channel, which may occur when they flow horizontally.

To-and-fro system

In this system, as the name implies, gas moves to and fro between the horse's lungs and the reservoir bag, through a canister filled with soda lime (Figure 4.3). The system is relatively simple and easy to maintain as it contains no valves; it is also the most portable type of large-animal breathing circuit. It has the disadvantage that the absorbent is used up from one end of the canister only and the dead space (in which no gas exchange occurs) increases during use. In order to keep dead space to a minimum the canister must be connected close to the horse's mouth, with the risk that soda lime dust be inhaled. It is more difficult to manage with a horse in dorsal recumbency as the canister must be supported above the surface on which the horse is lying.

The to-and-fro system is ideally suited for situations where equipment must be regularly transported between sites and for field anaesthesia entailing relatively minor surgery. It is less well suited to use in an operating theatre, where a mobile trolley with a circle system is more convenient.

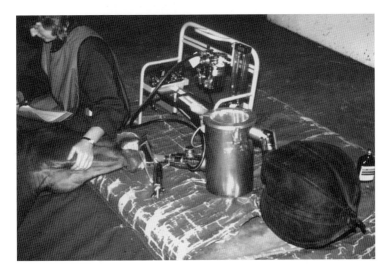

FIG 4.3 To-and-fro breathing circuit. (Courtesy of Dr JC Brearley.)

Circle system

This system is connected to the ETT by a Y-piece and the gases travel in one direction round a circle of tubing directed by valves in the expiratory and inspiratory limbs (Figure 4.4). The equipment is more complex than the to-and-fro system, and the valves require careful maintenance. Complex systems

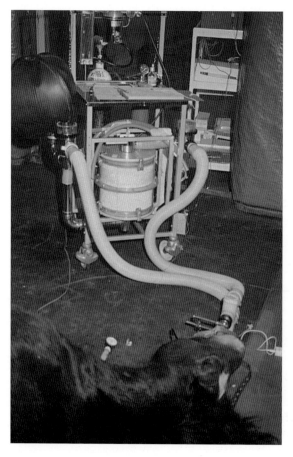

FIG 4.4 Circle breathing system.

where the circuit is incorporated into an anaesthetic trolley are convenient for regular use in an operating theatre, but simple adaptations of a to-and-fro system, by the addition of valves, breathing tubes and a Y-piece, function on the same principle. The circle is more efficient than the to-and-fro system as gases are continuously pushed in one direction through the absorbent, so it all contributes to carbon dioxide extraction. The canister is at some distance from the patient, which is easier to manage and prevents any absorbent dust entering the airway. The canister and valves are often mounted on the anaesthetic trolley, making the system compact and easily moved around a theatre. The internal volume of the circle system is much greater than that of a to-and-fro and gas concentrations change more slowly in response to alterations in gas flow rate or vaporiser setting.

GAS SUPPLY

The 'carrier gas' for the volatile agent should contain a minimum of 50% oxygen, and usually more. Most commonly oxygen alone is used as the carrier, but it can be combined either with nitrous oxide (pages 59–60) or with compressed 'medical' air; the flow rates of the individual gases are adjusted to achieve the required inspired oxygen concentration.

Oxygen is supplied to the breathing circuit from a 'low-pressure' source (60 psi, 4.1×10^3 kPa) on the anaesthetic machine. This in turn has come from high-pressure (1980 psi, 136.5×10^3 kPa) cylinders (small ones on the anaesthetic machine or via a pipeline from large cylinders) via a regulator that drops the pressure to 60 psi (4.1×10^3 kPa). Generators, which concentrate atmospheric oxygen, have been used to provide the anaesthetic carrier gas, but these are electrically driven and the maximum flow rate from the units currently marketed for veterinary use is inadequate for emergency use, so a cylinder source for 'back up' is still required. Oxygen is supplied to the breathing circuit at a flow rate sufficient to carry enough anaesthetic agent and to provide metabolic oxygen requirements. Flow rate is controlled by a flowmeter on the anaesthetic machine. The pressure in the breathing circuit remains close to atmospheric, either because excess gas is lost through an open 'pop-off' spill valve or because fresh gas flow is maintained at a rate sufficient to replace the metabolised oxygen (approximately 3–5 mL/kg/min). The circuit must not be connected in such a way that the 60 psi (4.1×10^3 kPa) pressure is directly transmitted to the lungs, as this causes barotrauma and may be fatal. In practice this means that fresh gas flow is adjusted sufficient to keep the rebreathing bag inflated.

Nitrous oxide, if used, is supplied in the same way as oxygen, from pipeline or cylinder, and the rate controlled by a flowmeter. It should not be used without a low oxygen pressure alarm that automatically cuts off the supply of nitrous oxide when the oxygen supply fails.

Air (medical) is supplied in the same way as oxygen. A low oxygen pressure alarm should also be incorporated, as the 20% oxygen in air is inadequate for the anaesthetised horse.

VAPORISER

Oxygen (and air or nitrous oxide if used) is passed from the flowmeter through the vaporiser containing the anaesthetic liquid. The gas thus carries the anaesthetic, now vaporised, to the breathing circuit. Precision vaporisers are designed to provide a constant concentration of anaesthetic agent at each setting in spite of changes in flow rate and temperature. Modern vaporisers, which must be serviced according to the manufacturer's instructions, are accurate over a wide range of gas flow rates. However, they are designed for use in human operating theatres and their temperature compensation is less good outside the range 18–35°C, so they may be particularly inaccurate at the lower temperatures often encountered with equine anaesthesia. The setting on the vaporiser is only tenuously related to the inspired anaesthetic concentration in the circuit, as the gases leaving the vaporiser are diluted by whatever is already in the circuit and the horse's lungs. Even the inspired concentration may not relate closely to the depth of anaesthesia, as this is dependent on the alveolar concentration whose relationship with the inspired is complex.

VENTILATOR

Ventilators suitable for use in horses all depend on replacing the reservoir bag of the breathing circuit with a 'bag-in-bottle' system that is used to squeeze the bag mechanically (Figure 4.5). Manual compression of the bag serves the same purpose. Ventilators are usually driven pneumatically, although some are controlled electrically. Provision for failure of the electrical supply must be made if an electrical system is used. The bottle section of the 'bag-in-bottle' system is gas tight and the bag acts as the rebreathing bag. The lungs are inflated when pressure in the bottle is increased, thereby squeezing the bag.

Separate ventilator trolleys are often used, simply attaching the ventilator bag in place of the reservoir bag used during spontaneous ventilation.

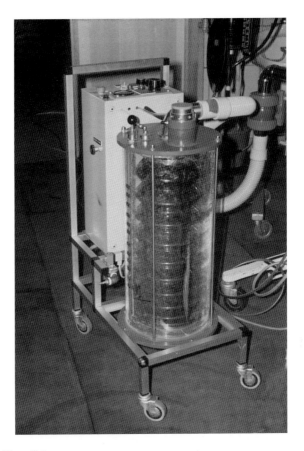

FIG 4.5   Bag-in-bottle ventilator.

Alternatively, complete trolleys incorporating ventilator, circle and rebreathing bag can also be used; in this case during spontaneous ventilation the same rebreathing bag is used, but with the bottle opened to atmosphere.

Any ventilator generally allows both volume and pressure to be regulated and must have a pressure-limiting device to prevent barotrauma to the lungs. Large-animal ventilators are complex and must be regularly maintained.

WASTE GAS SCAVENGING

Scavenging waste gases from large-animal rebreathing systems is relatively straightforward. The expired gases spilled through the 'pop-off' valve are directed by lightweight tubing (Figure 4.6) out of the operating theatre or into an activated-charcoal canister (Figure 4.7). An activated-charcoal system

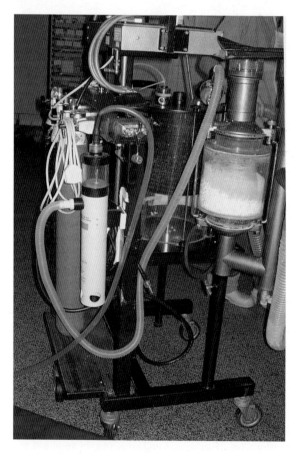

FIG 4.6   Waste gases expelled from the relief or 'pop-off' valve in the breathing circuit are collected into tubing and ducted away from the anaesthetic machine via an air brake.

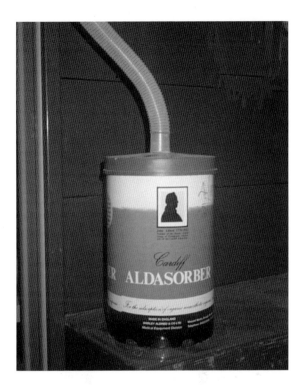

FIG 4.7   Activated charcoal canisters can be used to scavenge volatile anaesthetic agents but not nitrous oxide. They must be weighed regularly in order to detect exhaustion.

absorbs only volatile agents and does not remove nitrous oxide. It is essential that the charcoal is weighed on a regular basis and replaced when its absorption capacity is exhausted. Waste gas can be removed from the breathing system either actively by a pump, or passively, relying on the force of expiration by the animal. Active scavenging is more efficient and a number of commercial systems are now available. Such systems require the incorporation of an 'air brake' (Figure 4.6) to prevent the suction from the scavenging unit from emptying the rebreathing bag. Passive scavenging is simple to install but less reliable; if there is a hole in the system waste gas will leak back into the operating theatre as easily as it will travel through the intended route outside.

A more difficult area to scavenge is the recovery box, where anaesthetic agents may accumulate as the horse recovers. Exposure of staff to the agent becomes a consideration if assisted recoveries are routinely carried out. Health and safety regulations in most countries demand that exposure levels of anaesthetic agents are checked at regular intervals. The most common method is that staff wear badges for an operating session; the badges are then sent away for analysis. A risk assessment should be carried out for any pregnant members of staff.

PREPARATION OF THE ANAESTHETIC EQUIPMENT

All equipment should be checked carefully prior to use, so that everything is ready for connection as soon as to the horse becomes recumbent after receiving the intravenous agents.

Checks should include the following.

ENDOTRACHEAL TUBES

1. Two tubes should be available, one of the anticipated size and one smaller, in case of problems.
2. The cuff should be checked to ensure it does not leak. Cuffs should be left inflated for at least 5–10 minutes to ensure there is no slow leak (Figure 4.8). This is especially important if using IPPV, and before colic cases which may regurgitate during anaesthesia, as inhalation of gut material can lead to fatal respiratory complications.
3. Suitable connectors to attach the tube to the machine must be available.

THE ANAESTHETIC MACHINE

1. 'Full' and 'in use' cylinders must be checked for content and for lack of leaks.
2. The oxygen flowmeter is turned on (and off again) to ensure that oxygen flows and the meter does not stick.
3. Correct positioning of the vaporiser is confirmed, also that it is filled with the correct agent and can be turned on. Where a 'selectatec' system is used the vaporiser must be correctly locked on to the back bar.
4. The canister must contain fresh carbon dioxide absorbent.
5. The circle system must be correctly assembled, with the valves present and correctly positioned. Discs in 'turret' valves need to be checked to ensure

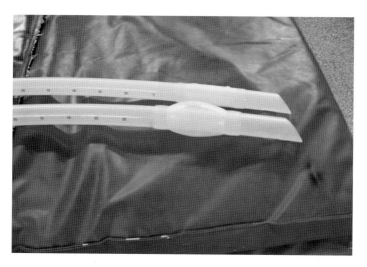

FIG 4.8 Cuffs are left inflated for at least 5–10 minutes before use to ensure there is no slow puncture.

that they are present and correctly seated. In some machines without turret valves it is possible to position the valves the wrong way round. Faults with valves mean the horse rebreathes in and out of the rebreathing bag without gas going through the absorbent, so inspired and expired carbon dioxide rise rapidly and the horse may appear to be waking up.

6. The circle system is checked for leaks. It is closed at the Y-piece and at the pop-off valve, the bag is filled with oxygen, and the system is tested by gently squeezing the bag (there should be no leaks). Additionally, the bag is left for 10 minutes to see that it does not deflate in this time.

PRACTICAL ADMINISTRATION OF INHALATION ANAESTHESIA

INDUCTION AND TRANSITION TO VOLATILE AGENT ANAESTHESIA

In adult horses the volatile agent is administered after induction of anaesthesia with an IV agent. The course of transition to maintenance of anaesthesia with the volatile agent will depend on the premedication and induction agents used. In general, α_2-agonist–ketamine induction (pages 34–37) allows more time than guaiphenesin–thiopental induction (pages 40–41). However, in all cases, further small doses of induction agent can be given to smooth the transition if anaesthesia becomes too light.

Inspired concentrations of 2–3% isoflurane (vaporiser setting around 4%) are given for the first 5–10 minutes to increase alveolar concentration rapidly. The inspired concentration is then gradually reduced to 1.3–1.6% (vaporiser setting around 2.5–3%) for maintenance. Isoflurane-induced respiratory depression may slow induction, and indeed it may prove necessary to ventilate. However, myocardial depression is severe if high doses are given, and it is better to be patient than to overdose. It is unwise to use a vaporiser setting higher than 5% isoflurane. Halothane is used in the same way as isoflurane; despite the lower MAC, its slower uptake and redistribution to fat compensate.

It is most common to use a high fresh gas flow (e.g. 8–10 L/min) during the first 10–15 minutes of anaesthesia in an adult horse. During this time the pop-off valve is open and excess gas flushed out of the circuit. The high flow rate enables more anaesthetic gas to be supplied to the circuit during induction and helps to flush nitrogen out of the horse's lungs and the circuit. After the initial period of high fresh gas flow the rate can be reduced to supply maintenance levels only. If nitrous oxide is used, oxygen flow rate must remain at least three times the metabolic oxygen consumption (i.e. 10 mL/kg/min) and the nitrous oxide:oxygen ratio should not fall below 50:50.

WHICH VOLATILE AGENT?
Isoflurane or halothane?

A recent epidemiological survey compared isoflurane and halothane in equine anaesthesia and demonstrated that there was no difference in overall death rate whichever agent was used. However, fewer horses receiving isoflurane died of intraoperative cardiac arrest, and in the 2–5-year age group fewer isoflurane horses died overall. Hypotension is similar with the two agents, but cardiac output is better maintained with isoflurane. Peripheral vasodilation in the presence of better cardiac output may lead to better muscle perfusion under isoflurane, but the complication of postanaesthetic myopathy appears equal with both agents. Respiratory depression is worse with isoflurane, making it difficult to maintain a stable plane of anaesthesia if the horse is not ventilated. Myocardial sensitisation to catecholamines is considerably less with isoflurane, and the lack of hepatic metabolism must make it a safer drug for the anaesthetist. A number of horses undergo a violent recovery from isoflurane, but the epidemiological survey demonstrated that this did not increase the number of fractures that occurred.

In human anaesthesia halothane is being superseded by the newer agents; it is no longer manufactured in the USA and is becoming difficult to obtain in many countries.

Sevoflurane and desflurane

Sevoflurane has been used successfully under clinical conditions in horses and is gaining popularity in the USA, Japan and some European clinics. Its low blood solubility leads to rapid induction, and many advocate the use of sedation in recovery, which is also fast. As with all volatile agents, however, cardiorespiratory depression is a significant feature of sevoflurane anaesthesia.

Published trials detailing clinical experience with desflurane are limited, but anecdotal reports from those who use it suggest that the ease of stabilisation of anaesthesia, coupled with the speed and completeness of recovery, make it an excellent agent for use in the horse. Cardiopulmonary changes are similar or less than with isoflurane, suggesting that desflurane may prove to be ideal for horses.

Nitrous oxide?

Many anaesthetists never use nitrous oxide in horses because of the dangers of hypoxia during or after anaesthesia, as discussed above (pages 59–60). However, it is an excellent analgesic and its use reduces the required concentrations of the more cardiopulmonary-depressant volatile anaesthetic agents. Its kinetics are useful in speeding the transition from intravenous to inhalation anaesthesia. However, the dangers of hypoxia are such that it should only be used with equipment that includes a system that cuts off nitrous oxide if the oxygen supply should fail. It is also undoubtedly safer to use if the inspired oxygen concentration can be measured, as well as arterial oxygen tension or saturation (pages 99–102). Specific contraindications to the use of nitrous oxide are cases where its ability to move into gas-filled spaces will cause exceptional problems, such as pneumothorax or in colic.

INTERMITTENT POSITIVE-PRESSURE VENTILATION (IPPV)

The decision to ventilate an anaesthetised horse is often a personal one but should take into account the range of effects on the body. There used to be a greater tendency to ventilate horses in the USA than in Europe. However, because a number of studies have indicated that a degree of hypercapnia may be beneficial (pages 136–137), hypercapnia is tolerated more readily. If no means of measuring arterial carbon dioxide or end-tidal carbon dioxide is available (Chapter 5), it is difficult to decide when ventilation is required.

A horse that is breathing slowly and erratically is often difficult to keep anaesthetised, and the decision to ventilate may be based on the need to achieve an even plane of anaesthesia rather than on the carbon dioxide retention. A horse breathing at 4 per minute or less is probably better ventilated. Equally, if it can be measured, a horse whose arterial carbon dioxide has reached 75 mmHg (10 kPa) probably should be ventilated. Hypercapnia tends to increase during anaesthesia, and if a long anaesthetic is anticipated it may be easier to ventilate from the start, rather than wait until hypercapnia becomes severe and upset the *status quo* by starting to ventilate later.

IPPV inevitably reduces cardiac output and decreases blood pressure. This is largely because during inspiration positive pressures replace the negative pressures that develop during spontaneous respiration. With spontaneous respiration, at inspiration, negative (relative to atmosphere) pressures draw blood into the thorax and increase venous return; this increases cardiac output according to the Frank–Starling mechanism. However, positive pressure restricts venous return and may have a marked effect on cardiac output and arterial blood pressure in the anaesthetised horse. Reduction of the arterial carbon dioxide tension also contributes to hypotension.

Once the decision to ventilate is made, the technique using a 'bag-in-bottle' system is straightforward. Most horses can be ventilated with peak pressures of 20–25 cmH$_2$O, a tidal volume of 1 L/100 kg and a rate of 6–8/min. Inspiratory pressure should be kept as low as is compatible with adequate volume. Ideally, ventilation is fine-tuned with further adjustment of volume and rate according to blood gas or end-tidal carbon dioxide measurements. Higher pressures may be required if the abdomen is distended. Unexpectedly high pressures must be investigated; they may mean that the airway is obstructed. Pressures should not exceed 60 cmH$_2$O or the lungs may be damaged. Arterial $PaCO_2$ should not be reduced below 40 mmHg (5.3 kPa) as this will reduce tissue perfusion. It is better to allow a degree of hypercapnia, and maintaining $PaCO_2$ in the low to mid-50s mmHg is perfectly acceptable.

Theoretically, it should be possible to assist ventilation rather than override the horse's own respiratory drive completely. Some ventilators have an 'assist' mode, in which the slight fall in pressure at the start of inspiration triggers an inspiration from the ventilator; such ventilators are usually set so as to intervene if the horse is apnoeic or bradypnoeic. Manual ventilation can be used, and intermittent support in this way is often sufficient to manage periods of inadequate spontaneous respiration. However, this is tedious if required frequently during long periods of anaesthesia.

ADJUNCTS TO MAINTENANCE OF VOLATILE ANAESTHESIA

The problems that may occur during any equine anaesthetic, inhalation or intravenous, are discussed in detail in Chapter 7. Two of the requirements of anaesthesia are interrelated: preventing response to noxious stimulation, and maintenance of adequate blood pressure. It can be surprisingly difficult to assess the depth of anaesthesia in horses; response to surgery can be sudden and violent. Response to hindlimb surgery in particular can occur even when anaesthesia is very deep, and probably results from direct spinal reflexes. Hypotension occurs in a dose–response manner with all volatile agents. Anything able to reduce the amount of volatile agent is likely to improve cardiovascular function.

PROVISION OF ADDITIONAL INTRAOPERATIVE ANALGESIA
Local anaesthesia
Local anaesthesia prevents noxious input from surgery and should be used wherever practical. The duration of effect depends on the anaesthetic used: long-acting analgesics such as bupivacaine and ropivacaine will extend analgesia into the recovery period. Specific local analgesic blocks for limbs and the head are well described for horses (see Chapter 6), but where such a block is not practicable local infiltration should be considered. Local analgesics can be added to the flushing fluids for arthrosocopy, or instilled into the joint at the end of surgery.

Bolus intravenous or intramuscular injections

A number of sedative, analgesic and anaesthetic agents injections have been advocated for bolus use when anaesthesia becomes light. These include the following:

- **Ketamine** (0.1–0.2 mg/kg) is the most successful as it has little effect on the cardiovascular system and has a fast onset of action. It may cause transitory apnoea. If repeated doses are required the total dose of increments should not exceed 2 mg/kg, and the last dose should preferably be given at least 10 minutes before the end of anaesthesia.
- **Diazepam** (0.02–0.04 mg/kg) has variable success and is usually used when trying to avoid giving more ketamine. It should not be given within at least 20 minutes of the end of anaesthesia as it may cause additional ataxia.
- **Opioids**
  - **Butorphanol** (0.02–0.04 mg/kg). Since opioids cause excitement they do not always increase the depth of anaesthesia. However, by providing underlying analgesia, butorphanol may improve the quality of anaesthesia in some circumstances; it may be more effective if given as premedication.
  - **Morphine** (0.1–0.2 mg/kg). As with butorphanol, there is some question whether morphine improves the quality of anaesthesia in horses. However, in most cases the additional analgesia may prevent response to a noxious stimulus. Repeated doses may lead to excitement during recovery (see Chapter 6).
- **Thiopental** (0.5–1.0 mg/kg) undoubtedly causes some further hypotension and may cause apnoea. However, it is effective in deepening anaesthesia quickly.
- **α_2 Agonists**
  - **Xylazine** (0.1–0.2 mg/kg). This should be given very slowly, as on occasions it may cause severe bradycardia or even transient cardiac standstill. As xylazine is relatively short acting and non-cumulative, doses can be repeated as required, but the total dose in any one hour is best limited to 0.5 mg/kg.
  - **Detomidine** (0.005 mg/kg IV or 0.005–0.01 mg/kg IM). Intravenous administration should be slow, which is difficult with the small volume of drug used. The IM route is recommended, as volumes are then more practicable; severe bradycardia is avoided; efficacy is obvious within 5–10 minutes, and the recommended doses are effective for about 1 hour. It is a suitable technique to use when the effect of the induction dose

of α_2 agonist has waned. The total dose should preferably not exceed 0.01 mg/kg/h. If IM detomidine is given within 30 minutes of the end of surgery, it may also provide sedation for recovery.

Infusions

Infusions of short-acting agents are preferable to bolus injections as they result in a steady state of anaesthesia and analgesia. Agents that have been used in this way include:

- **α_2 Agonists**
  - **Detomidine**. Infusions of 0.18 µg/kg/min have been shown markedly to reduce the amount of volatile agent used, with no serious side effects (page 23).
  - **Medetomidine** (3.5 µg/kg/min). Although medetomidine is not licensed for horses, there is now a great deal of experience of its use by infusion during anaesthesia. Medetomidine has potent analgesic properties and markedly reduces the dose of volatile agent required. Medetomidine is non-cumulative in the horse, even after infusions of 4 hours, and recovery from anaesthesia is rapid and calm after the infusion is stopped. The bladder must be catheterised and adequate fluid infused to replace the medetomidine-induced high urinary output.
  - **Xylazine** (0.035 mg/kg/min). There is surprisingly little information relating to xylazine infusion during volatile agent anaesthesia, although, like medetomidine, it is short-acting and provides good analgesia. The above infusion rate has been satisfactorily used as part of TIVA regimens.
- **Lidocaine:** 1–2 mg/kg over 15 minutes, then 0.05 mg/kg/min. Lidocaine infusions at the above doses reduce the required dose of volatile agents and are now widely used as an adjunct to inhalation anaesthesia. However, there is evidence that its use increases ataxia in recovery, so the infusion should be stopped 30 minutes before the end of anaesthesia. Half-litre bags of 0.2% (2 mg/mL) lidocaine are available commercially.

PREVENTION OR TREATMENT OF HYPOTENSION

Reduce the amount of volatile agent

Extra anaesthesia and analgesia can be provided by the methods listed above.

Infuse balanced electrolyte solution

Lactated Ringer's solution at 10 mL/kg/h increases venous return and helps to support blood pressure by enhancing cardiac output. The effect is short-lived, as the fluid leaves the circulation for other extracellular fluid (ECF) spaces, and so must be infused throughout anaesthesia. During prolonged surgery in normovolaemic and normotensive horses the rate of fluid administration should be reduced to prevent peripheral oedema.

Infuse inotropes

This is a popular and effective technique but should be employed only in addition to electrolyte infusion to ensure that the heart is able to fill adequately. The inotrope increases cardiac contractility, thereby increasing cardiac output and arterial blood pressure.

Dobutamine (0.25–5.0 μg/kg/min). Dobutamine is most conveniently made up by diluting 10 mL of concentrated solution (usually purchased as 250 mg in 20 mL) in 500 mL 5% dextrose, giving a solution containing 250 μg/mL. It is then given by continuous infusion, (e.g. for a 500 kg horse give 250 μg/mL infused at 30–600 mL/h). An infusion pump is useful but not essential. However, care must be taken when the electrolyte infusion rate is changed or stopped, as this will affect the inotrope infusion rate if the same catheter is used.

Dobutamine is a β_1-adrenergic agonist that increases cardiac contractility with little effect on heart rate, except at high doses when dysrhythmias may also occur. Increased contractility causes cardiac output to rise, which in turn leads to increased blood pressure. At high doses, increased peripheral resistance may also contribute to the rise in blood pressure. The effect on cardiac output and arterial blood pressure is dose dependent: around 0.25–1.0 μg/kg/min are usually sufficient, and low doses should be given initially and only increased if necessary. Dobutamine is also a positive chronotrope, but in horses an unexpected reflex bradycardia may occur; this is usually resolved if the infusion is slowed. Tachycardia and hypertension may occur if anticholinergics are given concurrently (pages 29–30). Dobutamine has a very short half-life and must be given by infusion for as long as the effect is required. It should not be stopped before the volatile agent administration is turned off.

Dopamine (0.25–5.0 μg/kg/min). Dopamine is conveniently made up in the same way as dobutamine and can again be given with an infusion pump, although this is not essential. The same care with concurrent infusions is required.

Dopamine has more complex dose-dependent actions than dobutamine and may increase cardiac output without an increase in blood pressure, making it more difficult to use to effect. Again, high doses may cause dysrhythmias. Dopamine has a very short half-life and must also be given by infusion for as long as its effect is required.

Ephedrine (0.03–0.1 mg/kg, single injection). Ephedrine is very effective in raising blood pressure as it increases cardiac contractility and causes peripheral vasoconstriction. The effect lasts for at least 30 minutes. However, ephedrine may not improve perfusion as much as a pure inotrope, and repeated doses are best avoided. Dobutamine is a better first choice.

Dopexamine. Dopexamine, a newer synthetic sympathomimetic, appears highly effective at improving cardiovascular function in the anaesthetised horse, but the side effects at the doses so far investigated render it unsuitable for clinical use.

Phenylephrine. Phenylephrine increases blood pressure through vasoconstriction. It has sometimes been used (0.02–0.04 mg/kg) to increase central blood pressure in anaesthetised horses. However, cardiac output and tissue perfusion are not improved and may decrease. It may have a place in severely hypotensive horses that fail to respond to inotropes such as dobutamine, but should not be the first line of treatment for hypotension.

Noradrenaline (Norepinephrine) is used in horses that are non-responsive to dobutamine, most commonly in animals undergoing surgery for colic. It is given to effect by infusion. A 1 mg/mL solution can be made up using 4 mL of 125 mg/mL commercial solution in 500 mL saline. The infusion rate should not exceed 6 mg/min (6 mL/min) in a 500 kg horse or vasoconstriction may be severe, to the extent of reducing cardiac output. Dobutamine is continued at the same time.

NEUROMUSCULAR BLOCKING AGENTS

Neuromuscular blocking agents have been used in human and small-animal anaesthesia for many years. They are used to improve operating conditions without increasing the dose of anaesthetic agent. Adequate or better relaxation is achieved with less cardiovascular depression, as anaesthesia sufficient only to induce unconsciousness is required. It appears that the dose of anaesthetic required is reduced further during neuromuscular blockade, as there is no tonic input from the muscle spindles. There are a number of situations in which neuromuscular blockade is of considerable value in equine anaesthesia (Chapter 7) and the development of modern short-acting, non-depolarising agents has made this possible.

Neuromuscular blocking agents should be used in horses only by those well experienced in equine anaesthesia. During neuromuscular blockade it is essential to ensure that the horse is anaesthetised, not simply paralysed. Anaesthetic administration must continue during paralysis. Increasing blood pressure, lacrimation and facial twitches are all signs of light anaesthesia and must receive prompt action. Neuromuscular blockade affects all skeletal muscles, including the muscles of respiration. It is thus essential that IPPV be provided throughout anaesthesia, using a mechanical ventilator.

Atracurium, a non-depolarising, competitive neuromuscular blocking agent is most commonly used in the horse. At normal body temperature and pH it breaks down spontaneously, so that cumulation is very unlikely. For short procedures a single dose of 0.2 mg/kg is given IV, which will give 10–15 minutes' relaxation. For longer procedures a loading dose of 0.2 mg/kg is given and then an infusion of 0.2 mg/kg/h is started. This should be stopped about 45 minutes before the anticipated completion of surgery.

Neuromuscular blockade should be monitored using train-of-four stimulation (Figure 4.9). This is more sensitive than a single twitch. Nerve stimulators that produce an appropriate intensity and duration of stimulation are available commercially. They are generally used on the facial or peroneal nerve,

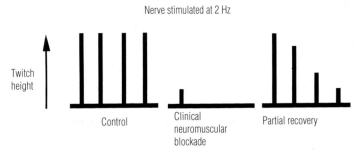

FIG 4.9   Train-of-four 'twitching' to monitor neuromuscular blockade.

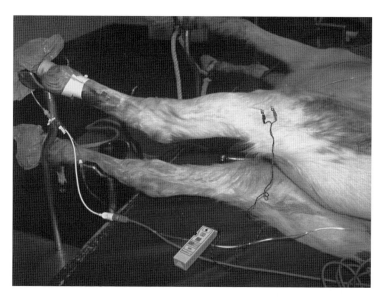

FIG 4.10 *Nerve stimulator used on the peroneal nerve to monitor neuromuscular blockade by train-of-four stimulation.*

depending on the surgical access required (Figure 4.10). A control train-of-four is assessed before the drug is given. The loading dose should reduce the response to a small first twitch, with the rest obliterated. Blockade should be maintained at this level as long as relaxation is required. The infusion is then turned off and pharmacological reversal can be started once all four twitches have returned. All four twitches should be back to control height before the horse is allowed to recover from anaesthesia. As a result of the spontaneous elimination of atracurium it may not be necessary to reverse the drug if anaesthesia is maintained for an hour or more after the infusion is turned off.

Neuromuscular blockade can be reversed if necessary 30–40 minutes after the last dose of atracurium is given or the infusion is turned off. All four twitches must be present, normally showing a marked decrease in height between the first and fourth twitches. Edrophonium is the drug of choice for reversal and can be given without anticholinergics. Incremental doses of 0.25–0.5 mg/kg are given to effect while the train-of-four and heart rate are monitored. Spontaneous respiration will return and must be back to full strength before the horse is allowed to recover from anaesthesia. Recovery after atracurium paralysis is usually calm and signs of weakness are absent. Rarely, inadequate reversal may lead to weakness when the horse tries to stand. It is not accompanied by excitement and responds favourably to a further small dose of edrophonium (around 0.1 mg/kg) and allowing the horse to stand in its own time.

Further reading

Clark L, Clutton RE, Blissitt KJ, Boller J, et al (2005) Effects of perioperative morphine administration during halothane anaesthesia in horses. *Veterinary Anaesthesia and Analgesia* **32**: 10–15.

Corley KTT (2004) Inotropes and vasopressors in adults and foals. *Veterinary Clinics of North America. Equine Practice* **20**: 77–106.

Grosenbaugh DA and Muir WW (1998) Cardiorespiratory effects of sevoflurane, isoflurane and halothane anesthesia in horses. *American Journal of Veterinary Research* **59**: 101–106.

Hall LW, Clarke KW and Trim CM (2001) *Veterinary Anaesthesia*, 10th edn. WB Saunders, London.

Johnston GM, Eastment JK, Taylor PM, et al (2004) Is isoflurane safer than halothane in equine anaesthesia? Results from a prospective multicentre randomised controlled trial. *Equine Veterinary Journal* **36**: 64–71.

Jones NY, Clarke KW and Clegg PD (1995) Desflurane – a new anaesthetic for the horse: a preliminary trial. *Veterinary Record* **137**: 618–620.

Kalchofner S, Ringer S, Boller J, et al (2005) Clinical assessment of anaesthesia with isoflurane and medetomidine in 300 equidae. Proceedings of the Association of Veterinary Anaesthetists, Rimini.

Matthews NS, Hartsfield SM, Carroll GL, et al (1999) Sevoflurane anaesthesia in clinical equine cases: maintenance and recovery. *Journal of Veterinary Anaesthesia* **26**: 13–17.

Muir WW and Hubbell JAE (1991) *Muir and Hubbell's Equine Anaesthesia: Monitoring and Emergency Therapy*. Mosby Year Book, St Louis.

Steffey EP, Woliner MJ, Puschner B and Galey FD (2005) Effects of desflurane and mode of ventilation on cardiovascular and respiratory functions and clinicopathologic variables in horses. *American Journal of Veterinary Research* **66**: 669–677.

Thurmon JC, Tranquilli WJ and Benson GJ (1996) *Lumb and Jones' Veterinary Anaesthesia*, 3rd edn. Williams & Wilkins, Baltimore.

Valverde A, Gunkelt C, Doherty TJ, et al (2005) Effect of a constant rate infusion of lidocaine on the quality of recovery from sevoflurane or isoflurane general anaesthesia in horses. *Equine Veterinary Journal* **37**: 559–564.

MONITORING

Monitoring means continuous surveillance of the anaesthetised horse. It is carried out to ensure that physiological function and the depth of anaesthesia are adequate. Abnormalities need to be detected as soon as they occur so that remedial action can be taken before a small change becomes a major problem. In horses anaesthetised with volatile agents the margin between surgical anaesthesia and overdose is small. In particular, the respiratory and cardio-vascular systems must be closely monitored. Measurements that can be made easily, such as pulse and respiratory rate, are used to infer information about the more fundamental physiological function of the cardiovascular and respiratory systems. A record should be kept of measurements made during anaesthesia (Figure 5.1). This enable trends to be seen and, should disaster occur, provides a record of what happened.

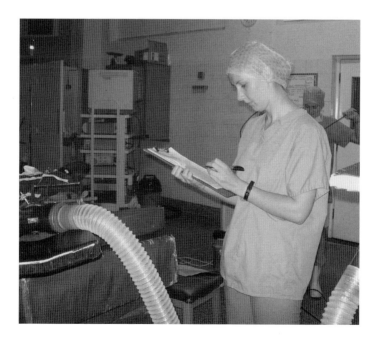

FIG 5.1   A written record should always be kept.

CARDIOVASCULAR SYSTEM

The aim during anaesthesia is to maintain adequate perfusion to all the tissues. Perfusion depends to a large part on the cardiac output. It is difficult to measure cardiac output during clinical anaesthesia and other factors are used to indicate, often indirectly, the state of tissue perfusion.

PULSE

The pulse should be regularly palpated (at least every 5 minutes) throughout anaesthesia. The horse is well supplied with superficial peripheral arteries: the facial, transverse facial, great metatarsal, common digital or digital arteries are all accessible (Figure 5.2). Pulse monitors such as the Doppler system used for indirect blood pressure monitors (Figure 5.6) can be used on the tail to indicate pulse rate and quality. Pulse oximetry (Figure 5.11) also acts as a peripheral pulse monitor.

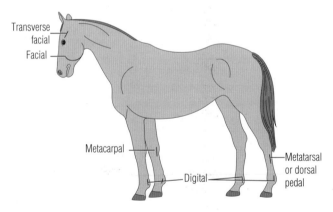

FIG 5.2 Superficial arteries suitable for pulse palpation or arterial catheter placement. The facial, transverse facial and dorsal pedal are the best for catheter placement.

Pulse quality provides information about peripheral circulation and, indirectly, about cardiac contractility. The palpated pulse depends on the difference between systolic and diastolic pressures (pulse pressure) and does not indicate blood pressure. Nevertheless, it is related to stroke volume, and a weak pulse is usually associated with hypotension. The pulse also feels weak with intense vasoconstriction, such as occurs immediately after an α_2 agonist or a catecholamine has been given, although in these cases blood pressure is high.

Pulse rate is usually remarkably stable in anaesthetised horses and changes very little in response to surgical stimulation. Movement or an increase in blood pressure is a more common response to inadequate anaesthesia. A hypovolaemic horse has a high pulse rate, which should decrease as the volume is replaced. Palpation of irregular beats indicates some form of dysrhythmia and should be investigated with the ECG.

MUCOUS MEMBRANES

Mucous membrane colour and capillary refill time give some guide to oxygenation and the adequacy of peripheral perfusion. The mouth is the best site to use in the horse. Refill time over 2 seconds is cause for concern, as it is associated with inadequate perfusion. Interpretation of colour is more subjective but gives a good, if approximate, guide to peripheral perfusion. However, hypoxaemia must be severe before cyanosis is seen, and should not be used as a low oxygen warning device!

The mucous membranes should be pink. Pale mucous membranes with a slow refill time and a slight grey tinge, often seen with halothane, presumably indicate less than adequate peripheral perfusion. A good healthy pink may indicate hypercapnia, but also indicates good perfusion. A toxic horse may have congested mucous membranes; improved colour is a sign of appropriate response to treatment and better peripheral perfusion. Grass-fed horses often have slightly yellow mucous membranes; this is related to the chlorophyll in the diet and should not be interpreted as jaundice unless there are accompanying signs of liver disease.

ARTERIAL BLOOD PRESSURE

Arterial blood pressure (ABP) provides a great deal of information about the adequacy of the cardiovascular system, and in addition to pulse and respiration is the most important aid to monitoring the anaesthetised horse. It should be used in all but the shortest field procedures and employed whenever volatile agents are used. ABP is related to, but not the same as, cardiac output (page 130). However, ABP provides invaluable indirect information about perfusion and has proved to be a robust means of monitoring the anaesthetised horse. ABP is also a monitor of depth of anaesthesia, as volatile agent-induced hypotension is dose dependent. A sharp increase in ABP may occur in response to surgery and usually marginally precedes movement when anaesthesia is too light.

The association between hypotension and myopathy (pages 139–146) is now well established. Mean ABP should be maintained at or above 70 mmHg, and as it is impossible to estimate ABP with any accuracy by simple clinical observation it must be measured, both to detect hypotension and to monitor the response to treatment. ABP can be measured either directly using a catheter in an artery or indirectly using a cuff and a peripheral pulse detector. The direct system is preferable as it gives a continuous record and is very easy to use in horses. Indirect systems are intermittent, depend on inflation of a cuff, and are more likely to fail in hypotension.

For direct ABP measurement a catheter is placed in an artery (Figure 5.3) and connected either to an aneroid manometer (Figure 5.4) or to a strain-gauge pressure transducer with amplifier and oscilloscope screen or paper trace (Figure 5.5). The aneroid system is simple and cheap but gives only mean arterial pressure. The electronic system is more expensive, but provides

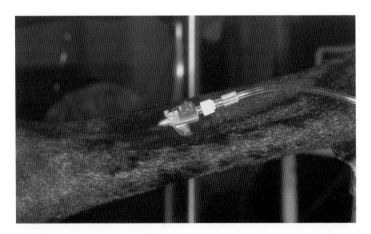

FIG 5.3 Catheter for arterial pressure measurement and blood sampling in the dorsal pedal artery – on the lateral side of the non-dependent hindlimb in a horse anaesthetised in lateral recumbency.

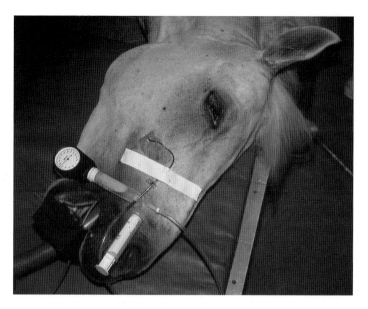

FIG 5.4   Direct blood pressure measurement using an aneroid manometer. The manometer should be raised level with the sternum to record blood pressure accurately. A 'butterfly' in the facial artery is used here for monitoring. Butterfly needles are easier to place than catheters but are easily dislodged and blocked. They are useful for short periods of blood pressure measurement and for gaining skill in placing arterial catheters.

systolic and diastolic pressures as well as a pulse waveform. Most modern systems integrate the waveform to give a mean arterial pressure. Systems developed for human anaesthesia, often incorporating an ECG, are suitable for use in horses.

The arterial catheter should be placed as soon as possible after induction: this should be a high priority, as serious hypotension may develop rapidly. A 22–20 swg 5 cm over-the-needle catheter is sufficient in most horses. Butterfly needles (see Figure 5.4) are easier to place and may be useful when a line is required quickly in a difficult artery, or when gaining experience of arterial catheterisation. Butterfly needles are, however, easily displaced and are not ideal when a long procedure is anticipated. Normal aseptic precautions are required and the catheter should be stitched or glued (cyanoacrylate

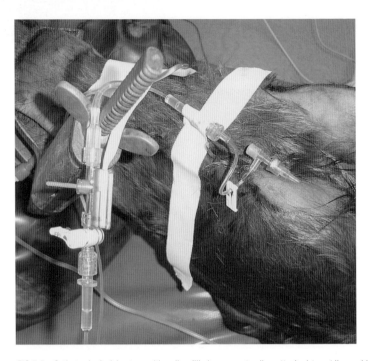

FIG 5.5a Catheter in facial artery with saline-filled manometer line attached to a 'disposable' strain-gauge transducer.

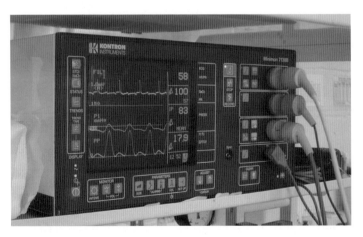

FIG 5.5b Amplifier and screen displaying arterial blood pressure waveform from pressure transducer. ECG and a pulse oximeter trace are also shown.

'superglue') to the skin. Extreme care should be taken not to drop any glue into the horse's eye when the facial or transverse facial arteries are used, and both catheter and glue must be removed carefully after use. The catheter should be flushed with heparinised saline and connected to stiff, saline-filled manometer tubing attached to the pressure transducer or manometer. The line should be flushed regularly (10–15-minute intervals) throughout anaesthesia. A continuous flush device is very useful and prevents occlusion of the arterial line, even in prolonged procedures.

Indirect methods use a cuff, usually placed around the tail, which is inflated above systolic pressure and then slowly deflated; systolic pressure is the cuff pressure at the first return of the pulse, usually detected by Doppler, with the detecting crystal distal to the cuff (Figure 5.6).

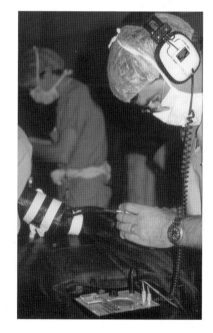

FIG 5.6   Doppler detection of pulse for indirect blood pressure measurement. The detector crystal is placed distal to the cuff on the tail. Headphones are used to help detect the return of pulse sounds as the cuff pressure is reduced.

Oscillometric methods also use a cuff to occlude the artery and depend on assessment of the pattern of pressure changes in the cuff. A number of automatic systems are available. The pressure in the cuff is raised above systolic and then allowed to fall; systolic, mean and diastolic pressures are automatically detected by the machine. Oscillometric equipment is generally designed for human or small-animal use and is not particularly reliable in horses.

The standard reference point for blood pressure measurements (venous and arterial) is the right atrium of the heart. With direct measurement of arterial blood pressure this is used simply by placing the transducer (electronic or aneroid) level with the atria. With non-invasive pressure, however, it becomes more difficult as the occluding cuff is the point at which the pressure is being measured, and can be considered as the transducer. With the horse in lateral recumbency a cuff on the tail will be close enough to the level of the heart for clinical accuracy. However, with a large horse in dorsal recumbency the cuff on the tail can be 20–40 cm (or even more) below the heart, resulting in blood pressure being measured as 20–40 cmH_2O (equal to approximately 15–30 mmHg) higher than is correct. Similarly, if the cuff is placed on the limb of a dorsally recumbent horse it will be well above the heart and the pressure as measured will be considerably lower than right atrial pressure. To correct pressures measured indirectly, the distance between the cuff and the heart should be measured in centimetres, the resulting measurement divided by 1.36 to convert it to mmHg (the specific gravity of mercury is 13.6), and the correction added (cuff above heart) or subtracted (cuff below heart) accordingly from the arterial pressure as measured.

THE ELECTROCARDIOGRAM (ECG)

The ECG provides information about the electrical activity of the heart; normal rhythm does not necessarily imply adequate cardiac output. Changes in rhythm or PQRS configuration may be associated with circulatory abnormalities and these cannot be diagnosed accurately without ECG recording. It is essential for any rational treatment that the nature of any dysrhythmia be identified. Changes in the ECG configuration may indicate systemic abnormalities: for instance, the T wave may change with hypoxaemia or electrolyte disturbances. Atrial fibrillation occasionally develops during anaesthesia (pages 131–132) and cannot be diagnosed without an ECG (Figure 5.7).

Commercially available ECG systems made for the medical profession are suitable for use in horses, although some alarm systems are persistently triggered

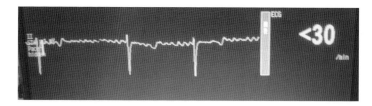

FIG 5.7   *Atrial fibrillation occasionally develops during anaesthesia and can only be diagnosed with any certainty using an ECG.*

by the horse's low heart rate. Precise location of the leads is not important as long as the axis is across the heart, as the main aim is to detect changes in ECG rhythm and configuration and not to make precise measurements. The leads may require placement according to surgical site, and a sternal–withers axis is often convenient in anaesthetised horses (Figure 5.8). Needles, crocodile clips or stick-on pads can all be used to attach electrodes (Figure 5.9).

The ECG should not be used without a waveform display as a heart rate monitor. The QRS-complex rate may remain remarkably constant even when the configuration has changed, there is no cardiac output and the horse is virtually dead.

CARDIAC OUTPUT

Lithium dilution techniques have made it possible to measure cardiac output under clinical conditions. A jugular catheter and an arterial sampling line are required. The system works on a simple dilution principle using lithium as the indicator, and has been extended to assess cardiac output using the pulse pressure contour with calibration by lithium dilution at intervals. Ketamine and most neuromuscular blocking agents interfere with measurement, and readings should not be taken immediately after administration of these compounds. Although consumables are not cheap, the system is practicable for clinical use.

Indication of cardiac output can be obtained from venous blood gases and capnography (see below).

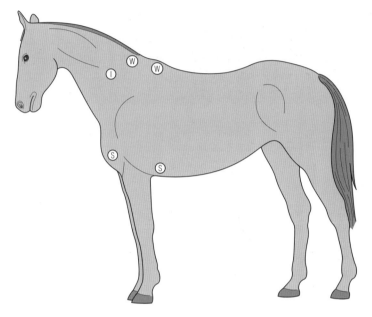

FIG 5.8   The ECG is adequately monitored during anaesthesia by leads placed in a 'sternal–withers' configuration. S, alternative sites for the sternal placement; W, alternative sites for the withers placement. I (indifferent) may be placed anywhere, but the neck is convenient. A good lead II trace is obtained with the 'right arm' lead placed at S and the 'left arm' lead at W and the 'left leg' lead at I. Many other lead configurations can be used as long as they span the heart.

RESPIRATORY SYSTEM

RESPIRATION

Respiratory movement of the chest wall and the rebreathing bag should be monitored regularly (at least every 5 minutes). It is important that both are watched, as disparity between the two indicates airway obstruction or disconnection. Low rates or apnoea can be detected, but it is difficult to tell from respiratory frequency and pattern alone whether ventilation is providing adequate gas exchange. A horse may appear to be breathing normally but be hypercapnic and hypoxaemic. More sophisticated equipment is required to

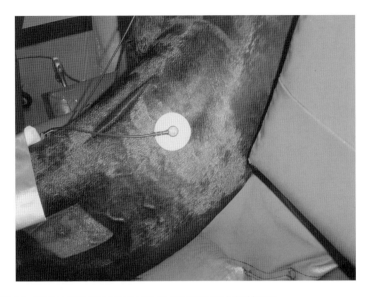

FIG 5.9 Stick-on ECG pads can be used on clipped or fine-haired horses.

provide information about carbon dioxide retention and oxygen haemoglobin saturation.

Respiratory frequency below 4 per minute is almost certain to be inadequate. However, 'periodic breathing', when the horse takes several breaths in a row and then none for 30–60 seconds, may be associated with surprisingly good gas exchange. Increased rate and depth of respiration may be seen with surgical stimulation and can be a useful guide to the depth of anaesthesia. Increased respiratory effort must be investigated; it is usually the first sign of airway obstruction. Cheyne–Stokes or gasping respiration suggests seriously deep anaesthesia, cardiovascular collapse and actual or impending death (pages 173–174), in spite of the apparent conscious movements that may accompany it.

END-TIDAL CARBON DIOXIDE MEASUREMENT (CAPNOGRAPHY)

End-tidal carbon dioxide is usually measured by infrared absorption. Commercially available capnographs made for the medical profession are

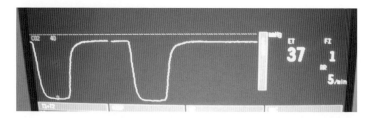

FIG 5.10 A normal capnogram; note the plateau at peak end-tidal carbon dioxide, and that trace returns to zero before inspiration. If the trace does not return to zero, valves and absorbents should be checked. In this example the end-tidal carbon dioxide is 37 mmHg. This lower-than-ideal value represents either overventilation (this horse was receiving IPPV) or could be an indication that cardiac output is low.

suitable for use in horses. Gases are sampled continuously from the endotracheal tube and the peak carbon dioxide concentration is taken as end-tidal alveolar concentration.

Capnography provides information that cannot be ascertained from simple clinical measurement and is a worthwhile investment for large equine clinics (Figure 5.10). An inspired reading of greater than 0 mmHg carbon dioxide indicates that the breathing circuit is not extracting all the carbon dioxide through exhausted absorbent or faulty valves; this must be investigated and remedied immediately.

End-tidal gas is effectively the same as alveolar gas, and the technique provides information about both gas exchange and the ability of the heart to pump blood to the lungs. In perfect lungs, arterial and end-tidal carbon dioxide are the same; however, in the anaesthetised horse arterial carbon dioxide is usually higher as a result of ventilation–perfusion mismatching. End-tidal carbon dioxide is thus only a guide to arterial carbon dioxide. If expired carbon dioxide is recorded continuously on a paper or oscilloscope trace, further information is supplied about lung function. Normal lungs produce a sharp rise then a plateau, but a slower rise without a plateau is seen in small airway disease.

High end-tidal carbon dioxide is seen when arterial carbon dioxide is high and gas exchange is good; it indicates that respiration is inadequate to excrete all the carbon dioxide being produced. Anaesthetic-induced respiratory depression is the commonest cause, but high arterial carbon dioxide is also seen when bicarbonate has been used to treat a metabolic acidosis, leading to carbon dioxide production.

During IPPV when respiration is constant, capnography provides a monitor of the cardiovascular system. Low alveolar carbon dioxide indicates a low cardiac output as pulmonary perfusion is low. In this case arterial carbon dioxide is high and cardiac output is inadequate to pump blood to the lungs fast enough for carbon dioxide removal. In the same way, during spontaneous respiration low end-tidal carbon dioxide readings that appear incompatible with the ventilation are most likely a result of low cardiac output. Whether breathing is controlled or spontaneous, low end-tidal carbon dioxide readings must prompt immediate assessment of cardiovascular function and instigation of appropriate support (pages 130–131, 171–174).

PULSE OXIMETRY

Pulse oximetry is a non-invasive method of measuring blood oxygen–haemoglobin saturation and is thus an extremely sensitive way to detect changes in arterial oxygenation. It depends on passing two beams of different-wavelength red light through tissue; the light is differentially absorbed by saturated and unsaturated haemoglobin. The machine processes this information and calculates the saturation. Changes in pulsatile flow are detected, and the system also acts as a pulse monitor. Oximeter probes are placed on any non-pigmented area where light can be transmitted through the tissue. The tongue, non-pigmented lips and the nasal septum have proved most successful in horses (Figure 5.11). Most systems have been developed for use in humans and do not perform well in horses. However, models with probes adapted for this species are now available and are proving relatively robust. Pulse oximetry is useful in this species, as horses are likely to become hypoxaemic even when breathing high oxygen concentrations. Saturation should remain over 90%. An important and valuable attribute of the pulse oximeter is that it is a pulse detector and provides highly relevant information about the quality of peripheral perfusion.

Oxygen haemoglobin saturation falls either when the inspired oxygen concentration is inadequate or when pulmonary gas exchange is impaired. The machine's response is immediate, allowing rapid treatment. It is important

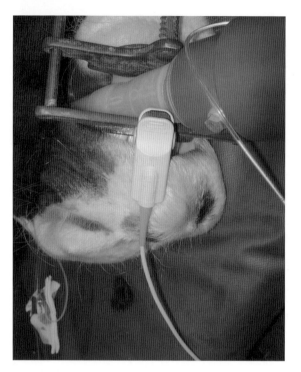

FIG 5.11 Pulse oximeters are commonly used on tongue or nasal septum, but often work well on a white lip.

to remember that pulse oximetry detects only oxygen saturation and is not affected by carbon dioxide. It cannot be used as a simple respiratory monitor. If breathing oxygen-enriched air a horse may be well oxygenated but still have sufficient respiratory depression to retain carbon dioxide. However, oxygen saturation over 90% in a horse breathing air probably indicates that respiration is adequate to remove carbon dioxide also.

BLOOD GAS ANALYSIS

Blood gas measurement no longer requires sophisticated, expensive equipment that needs careful maintenance. New portable systems with disposable cartridge electrodes are now commercially available, bringing the technology within reach of the private equine clinic.

Measurement of arterial blood oxygen and carbon dioxide tensions is fundamental for accurate assessment of pulmonary gas exchange. Adequate oxygen delivery and removal of carbon dioxide are essential, and oxygen supply and ventilation can be adjusted rationally if arterial gas tensions are known. The pH, also fundamental to normal homoeostasis, is traditionally measured with the same equipment.

Respiratory acidosis is common in the spontaneously breathing anaesthetised horse and can be treated by increasing ventilation to reduce arterial carbon dioxide. Metabolic acidosis may be seen in a horse with colic, and can only be detected and treated rationally if the pH can be measured. Alkalosis is extremely rare in the anaesthetised horse, but cannot be detected without blood gas measurement.

Mixed venous oxygen tension also provides information about perfusion. Values below 40 mmHg usually indicate that tissue perfusion is inadequate to meet demand and the tissues are extracting more of the supplied oxygen than normal. Mixed venous (pulmonary artery) samples are not easily obtained in clinical cases, but jugular samples are closely related and can be used in this way. The most information is gained if mixed venous and arterial blood samples are taken simultaneously: in this case, if the arterial value is normal or high (above 90 mmHg) and the venous value below 40 mmHg immediate assessment and support of the cardiovascular system is indicated. Venous samples taken from other sites cannot be used in this way as they relate only to perfusion of the area drained by the vein in question.

Blood gas measurement is performed on arterial or venous samples taken under anaerobic conditions. Arterial tensions may change very quickly, and these measurements are only useful in anaesthesia if they can be performed immediately after the sample is withdrawn.

INSPIRED OXYGEN CONCENTRATION
Virtually all anaesthesia for major surgery in horses is carried out using a rebreathing circuit. The oxygen concentration in the circuit is thus unknown, as the fresh gas is diluted by that already in the circuit. If nitrous oxide is used it becomes more critical to know the exact oxygen concentration because this may decrease as nitrous oxide accumulates in the circuit. The only reliable method of ensuring that the inspired oxygen concentration does not become too low is to measure it. A number of in-circuit oxygen

meters are commercially available, most based on the fuel-cell method. The standalone units are relatively cheap and serve a useful purpose as a safety device.

The exact inspired oxygen requirement depends on the individual horse; some may need close to 100% oxygen to ensure adequate arterial oxygenation. If oxygen saturation or tension cannot be measured, inspired oxygen concentration should be maintained at at least 50%.

DEPTH OF ANAESTHESIA

Measurement of the depth of anaesthesia depends almost entirely on indirect assessment of parameters that are dependent on CNS depression. Clinical observation is the mainstay, but indirect guides, particularly end-tidal anaesthetic concentrations, are invaluable. Clinical assessment of depth of anaesthesia is notoriously difficult in the horse, not helped by the way different drugs may alter cardinal signs.

Depth of anaesthesia depends on the procedure being performed. For instance, light anaesthesia is sufficient for non-painful diagnostic procedures but should be deeper for surgery. Ideally, the horse should just not move in response to noxious stimuli. A slight increase in respiration and sometimes a slight rise in blood pressure at the first incision indicate that the depth of anaesthesia is satisfactory.

EYE POSITION
Eye position provides some useful information as to the depth of anaesthesia. During volatile-agent anaesthesia nystagmus usually indicates that anaesthesia is too light for surgery. Unfortunately, however, this may also develop following cardiac arrest (page 173). At surgical depth at least one eye (position is often asymmetrical) is usually rotated forwards (Figure 5.12), and both should be closed and wet. An open, central, dry eye is seen when the horse has been overdosed.

ALVEOLAR CONCENTRATION OF ANAESTHETIC AGENT
Modern anaesthetic agent monitors, often combined with capnography, provide accurate measurement of inspired and expired anaesthetic agent concentrations.

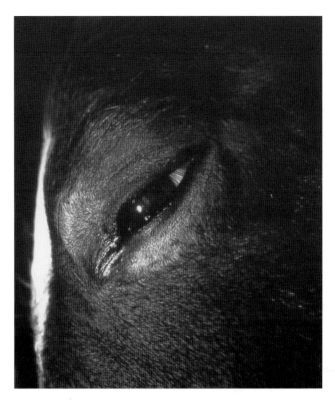

FIG 5.12 At a depth of anaesthesia suitable for surgery at least one of the eyes is usually rotated forwards so that a triangle of white sclera is seen. The eye is partially closed and wet from limited tear production.

Older infrared monitors suffer from interference by exhaled methane. Piezoelectric systems are accurate in horses as long as water vapour is excluded.

The inspired anaesthetic concentration bears little relation to the setting on the vaporiser when a rebreathing system is used, as the fresh gas flow is diluted by that already in the circuit. The end-tidal anaesthetic concentration is proportional to the brain concentration and hence to the depth of anaesthesia.

The dose of volatile agent required for surgery is reduced by other CNS depressants used concurrently and for premedication and induction. After common premedication and induction protocols alveolar concentrations of around 1.1–1.5 MAC (depending on the agent) are suitable for most surgical procedures, and measurement of end-tidal agent allows a constant concentration to be maintained.

NEUROMUSCULAR FUNCTION

Monitoring of neuromuscular function is described in Chapter 4, pages 82–83, in the section on neuromuscular blocking agents.

Further reading

Bhavani-Shankar Kodali. Capnography. A comprehensive educational website. www.capnography.com.

Hall LW, Clarke KW and Trim CM (2001) *Veterinary Anaesthesia*, 10th edn. WB Saunders, London.

Linton RA, Young LE, Marlin DJ, et al (2000) Cardiac output measured by lithium dilution, thermodilution, and transesophageal Doppler echocardiography in anesthetized horses. *American Journal of Veterinary Research* **61**: 731–737.

Moens Y (1989) Arterial-alveolar carbon dioxide tension difference and alveolar dead space in halothane anaesthetised horses. *Equine Veterinary Journal* **21**: 282–284.

Moens Y, Gootjes P and Lagerweij E (1989) The influence of methane on the infrared measurement of halothane in the horse. *Journal of Veterinary Anaesthesia* **18**: 4–7.

Muir WW and Hubbell JAE (eds) (1991) *Muir and Hubbell's Equine Anaesthesia: Monitoring and Emergency Therapy*. Mosby Year Book, St Louis, 153–179.

Taylor PM (1981) Techniques and clinical application of arterial blood pressure measurement in the horse. *Equine Veterinary Journal* **13**: 271–275.

Thurmon JC, Tranquilli WJ and Benson GJ (eds) (1996) *Lumb and Jones' Veterinary Anaesthesia*, 3rd edn. Williams & Wilkins, Baltimore, 409–424.

Whitehair KJ, Watney GC, Leith DE, et al (1990) Pulse oximetry in horses. *Veterinary Surgery* **19**: 243–248.

Young S (1989) Monitoring the anaesthetised horse. *Equine Veterinary Education* **1**: 45–49.

6

ANALGESIA

Equine analgesia has been somewhat neglected until relatively recently. However, it is now widely acknowledged that horses need good pain management, and a number of new techniques are in regular clinical use.

There is still some argument against analgesia in horses. A long-held belief is that if the pain of an injured body part is removed, the animal will overuse the part and cause further damage. This is unacceptable on humanitarian grounds and has limited foundation on practical grounds. Noxious stimuli cause effects in the spinal cord that correlate with the degree of stimulation. Limited input, leading to 'physiological pain', does not cause long-term effects and is essential for survival. More intense and prolonged stimulation, resulting from significant tissue damage, sensitises the nociceptive system causing 'clinical' pain. This process of sensitisation is known as 'wind-up'. Clinical pain is severe, easily provoked, and present even when the animal does not move. A horse experiencing this type of pain often becomes agitated and may cause more damage to the site of injury than one that is calm and relaxed as a result of good pain relief and physical support. Clinical pain may also contribute to a violent recovery from anaesthesia, potentially leading to self-inflicted trauma as well as damage to the surgical site.

Concern about the side effects of analgesics is another reason that they are withheld from horses. However, these side effects are always less significant in animals in pain than in normal individuals, particularly with the opioids. A further anxiety is that analgesia may mask a worsening disease condition, particularly infection. This is a real concern in a number of conditions in horses, most obviously in the treatment of infected joints and tendon sheaths, but should not preclude good pain management. Generally, as long as the overall condition of the animal is taken into account, the progress of the disease is not misdiagnosed as treatment progresses. As the condition improves the dose or frequency of analgesic treatment can be decreased and, if necessary, cover can be reduced briefly on a daily basis to assess the disease progress.

A third reason for reticence in the administration of analgesics is the difficulty of recognising when a horse is suffering pain. The horse is essentially a 'prey' animal and does not display behaviour that would make it appear vulnerable to a predator. Subtle signs of pain may be difficult to detect and interpret, and inappropriate anthropomorphism is all too easy. Signs of mental withdrawal, detachment, keeping very still, or, conversely, agitated restlessness, are all important behavioural signs indicating that a horse is in pain. General signs of suffering, with head down, ears slightly back and simple unwillingness to interact with people, are often a result of pain. Only violent behaviour in a horse with severe colic is easily recognised.

The benefits of good perioperative analgesia are obvious, not least as far as the welfare of the individual horse is concerned. Benefit also accrues because the adverse physiological effects of severe pain are considerable, and good pain relief may lead to better long-term outcome. Pain clearly affects a horse's general demeanour, and in particular its willingness to eat. Surgery and trauma lead to a substantial increase in energy requirements, as a result of the need for tissue repair. If this is not covered by an increase in energy intake, marked weight loss occurs and the immune system is impaired. Good pain relief often changes an injured horse's despondent inappetance and aids recovery.

The best pain management is provided by preventing the spinal cord sensitisation that leads to clinical pain. This is termed pre-emptive analgesia and depends on blocking or modulating incoming nociceptive signals, thereby preventing the sensitisation process from starting or progressing. The benefits of pre-emptive analgesia have been exploited in perioperative pain management in small animals and in humans, and are equally applicable to horses. A number of drugs can be used in this way, particularly opioids, N-methyl-D-aspartate (NMDA) antagonists such as ketamine, and α_2 agonists.

General anaesthesia, by its very nature, provides analgesia because the horse is unconscious. However, unless the anaesthetic protocol includes drugs that are themselves analgesics (i.e. would cause analgesia in the conscious animal), sensitisation still develops and postoperative pain will be severe when the horse regains consciousness; the neurons will still be sensitised even though the surgical stimulus has ceased. Postoperative analgesia will therefore be markedly improved if analgesics are used as part of the anaesthetic protocol. Following surgery there is also continued noxious input from the inflammation that develops at the surgical site, and further analgesic administration is still required postoperatively.

In general, perioperative administration of analgesics incurs the further benefit of reducing the required dose of anaesthetic used for induction and maintenance. Lidocaine, ketamine, the α_2 agonists and the opioids have this effect, although in horses the effect of opioids on anaesthetic requirements is complex (page 108).

A combination of different analgesic methods, 'multimodal analgesia', is most effective. Combinations of drugs that act via different mechanisms produce a synergistic, or at least additive, effect and have the advantage of enhanced analgesia without additional toxicity when the drugs are metabolised and excreted by separate routes.

OPIOIDS

Opioids are potent analgesics that act at a number of receptors, of which the μ receptor is responsible for the most potent analgesic effect. Activation of the μ receptor also causes side effects such as respiratory depression, locomotor stimulation and changes in gut motility. Other receptors (particularly κ, δ and σ) contribute some but less intense analgesia. Morphine, methadone, pethidine (meperidine) and fentanyl are agonists at the μ receptor and are subject to legislation controlling dangerous drugs. A number of synthetic opioids have varied agonist–antagonist actions at different receptors, depending partly on their dosage, and are sometimes subject to less stringent legal controls. Of these agents, butorphanol is often used in the horse. Buprenorphine, a longer-acting partial μ agonist, has more recently found a place in equine work. The μ-agonist opioids can be reversed by opiate antagonists such as naloxone, naltrexene and nalmefene. This is rarely required when normal therapeutic doses are used for chemical restraint or premedication, but valuable in an emergency. It is considerably more difficult to reverse the partial agonists.

Opioids are still the most widely accepted analgesic drugs, although their use in the horse is somewhat controversial. However, methadone and pethidine have been used in horses for several decades in Europe, and there is no doubt that opioids are effective in this species. Opioid-induced respiratory depression is not usually a problem, particularly when the drugs are used in small doses for chemical restraint.

Locomotor stimulation may cause difficulties, particularly with morphine. Excitatory phenomena are common in the normal, healthy research horse, and are generally seen as muscular twitching, particularly around the muzzle, as uncontrollable walking, or occasionally as a violent reaction. It is very rarely a problem in clinical cases that require pain relief, and when opioids are used in combination with sedatives (Table 2.1, page 29). Locomotor stimulation is dose dependent and the violent forms are more common following IV than IM injection. A further manifestation of opioid-induced excitation in horses is that, in contrast to at least dogs and humans, these drugs do not consistently reduce the minimum alveolar concentration (MAC) of volatile agent required to prevent purposeful movement in response to a specified stimulus. In horses MAC may actually be increased. Opioids do, however, increase the depth of anaesthesia as assessed by electroencephalography. This anomaly does not affect the clinical use of opioids, and most anaesthetists agree that the analgesic effect of perioperative opioids in horses is similar to that in other species.

A further complication from the use of opioids is the increased risk of postoperative colic, which has been reported by some centres. This is presumably a result of opioid-suppression of normal gut motility. Postoperative colic is more likely to occur with higher doses, and probably with prolonged systemic administration. However, the aetiology of postoperative colic is not fully understood; it is likely to be multifactorial, depending also on factors such as preoperative starvation and the administration of other drugs around the time of surgery.

The epidural route of administration can be used to provide analgesia with morphine whilst reducing the systemic effects. This may well be the route of choice for this drug, as its solubility characteristics are well suited for epidural administration. The method is described below (pages 117–120).

Morphine and methadone are generally given systemically at 0.1–0.12 mg/kg. Their effects last around 3–4 hours after IV or IM injection. Methadone is available as both the racemic mixture and the active L-isomer. Theoretically, the L-form should be twice as potent, but similar doses of both forms (in mg/kg) are widely used. Pethidine (1–2 mg/kg) given IM provides good analgesia with some sedation for 1–2 hours. It has a spasmolytic action on the gut and so is an excellent analgesic for spasmodic colic. Anaphylactoid reactions may occasionally occur if pethidine is given IV.

μ-agonist opioids are generally accepted as the best analgesics, but butorphanol (0.05–0.1 mg/kg, IM or IV), a κ-agonist opioid, is widely used in horses for pain relief and sedation. The degree of analgesia is often disappointing and also of very short duration. Butorphanol infusion (0.013 mg/kg/h) has been used to overcome the limited duration of action. This provides effective pain relief for many hours but may cause faecal impaction; output should be carefully monitored. Butorphanol has also been used by injection two to three times per day to provide several days' analgesia. This provides less effective pain relief than infusion, but although it reduces gut motility it does not usually cause impaction.

Fentanyl is a relatively short-acting potent μ-agonist opioid that has not been widely used in the horse. However, a patch formulation for transdermal administration has been used to provide pain relief of several days' duration to supplement NSAIDs when analgesia proved inadequate. One to three 150 μg patches are placed on clipped, thin skin inaccessible to the horse and are effective for around 3 days (Figure 6.1).

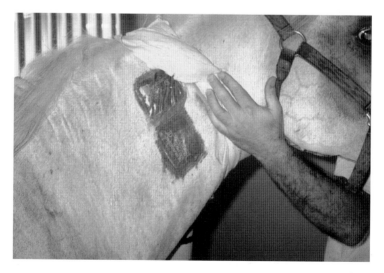

FIG 6.1 Fentanyl patches used to supply continuous analgesia through the transdermal route. Onset is slow, and other analgesic cover is required at this stage. Analgesic effect is variable and must be monitored throughout use. (Photograph courtesy of Dr NS Matthews.)

Buprenorphine is a partial μ-agonist opioid very widely used for pain relief in small animals. There is limited experience of buprenorphine in horses, but it has the advantage of providing much longer duration of analgesia than the other opioids and has considerable potential as an analgesic in this species. Anecdotal reports suggest that 0.005 and 0.010 mg/kg give many hours (>6) of analgesia.

NON-STEROIDAL ANTI-INFLAMMATORY DRUGS (NSAIDs)

NSAIDs provide excellent postoperative analgesia in the horse, probably both by a direct action and by reduction of inflammatory oedema. They are routinely given by injection before or during anaesthesia, so that they will be effective during the recovery period. Some preparations may affect the cardiovascular system, so IV administration should be slow, over at least 1 minute in the anaesthetised horse. Most NSAIDs inhibit prostaglandin synthesis, and in the dog their use during hypotensive anaesthesia has been associated with renal damage. Despite the fact that horses often develop marked hypotension during inhalation anaesthesia, no similar problems have been encountered in this species.

The NSAIDs are analgesic largely by virtue of their inhibition of cyclooxygenase (COX), which is responsible for production of inflammatory mediators, including the prostaglandins. Products of COX have a homoeostatic role in intestinal mucosal protection, renal autoregulation and maintenance of normal platelet function; hence COX inhibition has the potential to cause toxicity through one of these actions. However, NSAIDs have been used for many years in horses and there are few serious reports of toxicity when recommended doses are used. Postoperatively, careful monitoring of faecal output is essential as long-term use of higher doses may lead to overdose; the first sign of intestinal ulceration in horses is commonly diarrhoea.

There are at least two isoforms of COX: COX1, generally responsible for production of homoeostatic prostaglandins, and COX2, which is produced in large quantities in inflammation. It is likely that NSAIDs that selectively inhibit COX2 rather than COX1 may be less toxic. However, most of the studies to date relates to human or rat physiology, and the benefits or otherwise of COX2 inhibitors in horses is largely unknown.

Phenylbutazone and flunixin have been used for analgesia in horses for many years. Numerous newer NSAIDs have been used more recently, but there is no clear evidence that any provides obviously better analgesia than any other. The choice of NSAID for perioperative and long-term analgesic therapy is usually based on personal preference, the available routes of administration and cost. The benefit of using NSAIDs concurrently with opioids is generally borne out by widespread clinical experience.

LIDOCAINE INFUSION

Lidocaine infusions have been shown to reduce volatile anaesthetic requirements (page 79) and have been used to provide analgesia in conscious horses and during surgery for colic (loading dose of 1–2 mg/kg followed by infusion of 0.05 mg/kg/min). Lidocaine is prokinetic and is believed to enhance the return of intestinal activity after colic surgery. Lidocaine overdose leads to CNS effects and a potential for cardiac dysrhythmias, therefore careful monitoring is required.

LOCAL ANAESTHETIC BLOCKS

For surgery in locations where suitable nerve blocks can be carried out, local anaesthetic agents can be used to provide complete analgesia. This enables surgery in standing sedated horses or reduces the amount of general anaesthetic agents required. Local analgesics also provide excellent postoperative analgesia. Often it is practicable to perform specific nerve blocks (Figures 6.2, 6.3). Their use in limbs is limited to those affecting the knee, hock and below, as higher blocks may interfere with the horse's ability to stand. Blocks below carpus and hock rarely cause any problem for recovery. Where suitable specific regional blocks are not practicable, local infiltration or instillation still provides excellent pain relief (Figure 6.4). For instance, lidocaine has been added to flushing fluids used during the treatment of peritonitis.

Lidocaine is not usually used for precise nerve blocks in horses as it causes tissue oedema. However, where such reaction is not relevant, for example in local infiltration of a wide area, lidocaine is still suitable. Nevertheless, mepivacaine is the preferred agent. Where a prolonged effect is required, as for postoperative analgesia, long-acting agents such as bupivacaine (or ropivacaine) are required; some tissue swelling may result but is rarely a clinical problem.

Text continued on p. 114

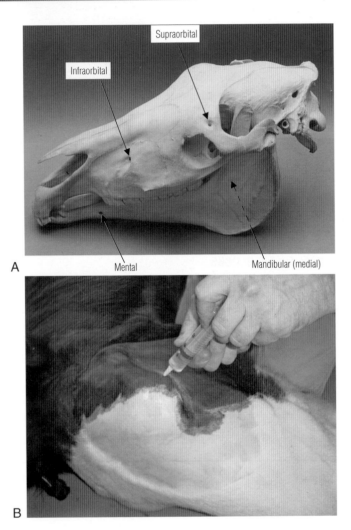

A
Infraorbital
Supraorbital
Mental
Mandibular (medial)

B

FIG 6.2 Local anaesthetic blocks around the head enable many surgical procedures to be performed in the standing horse. Given during general anaesthesia they reduce anaesthetic requirements and provide postoperative analgesia. (A) Points of injection for infraorbital, supraorbital, mental and mandibular nerve blocks. (B) A retrobulbar nerve block placed in the anaesthetised horse prior to surgery provides both perioperative analgesia and also reduces vagally induced cardiac dysrhythmias.

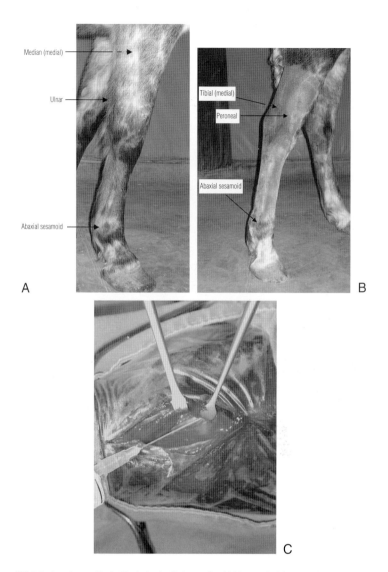

FIG 6.3a Local anaesthetic blocks in the limb are also highly practicable, providing both intra- and postoperative analgesia. (A) Points of injection in the forelimb. The abaxial sesamoid block is suitable for any foot surgery. Median and ulnar may be used for pain relief higher up the limb, including the carpus. (B) Hindlimb. Abaxial sesamoid as for forelimb. Tibial and peroneal may be used for pain relief higher up the limb, including the tarsus. (C) Local anaesthetic solution may be applied to any appropriate nerve that is exposed surgically.

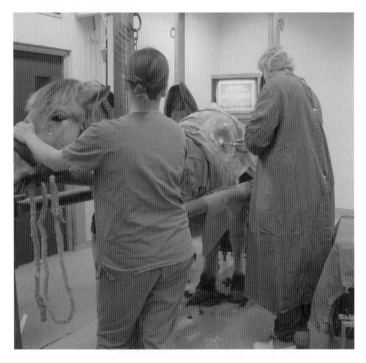

FIG 6.4 Local anaesthetic techniques for standing laparoscopic abdominal surgery can include regional methods such as paravertebral, but usually simple local infiltration is adequate. Analgesia for such surgery is also greatly enhanced with epidural morphine/detomidine (page 116).

α_2-ADRENOCEPTOR AGONISTS

It is well known that this group of drugs provides analgesia, particularly visceral. The analgesic effect is at least in part via the stimulation of α_2 receptors in the dorsal horn of the spinal cord. It is difficult to use these drugs for analgesia in the conscious horse, as sedation is inevitable. The use of α_2 agonists as part of premedication, or by infusion during anaesthesia (page 79), may contribute to postoperative analgesia. However, undoubtedly the most efficient way of using the analgesic effect of these drugs is via the epidural route. This is discussed below (pages 115–117).

KETAMINE

Ketamine, generally known as a dissociative anaesthetic, has been revisited as an analgesic by virtue of its action as an NMDA receptor antagonist in the spinal cord. Subanaesthetic doses appear to enhance postoperative analgesia. It is likely that the use of ketamine for induction and supplementation during maintenance of anaesthesia contributes to postoperative analgesia. Ketamine infusions have also been used to provide anaesthesia in conscious horses (0.4–0.8 mg/kg/h) for several days. There is some experience of ketamine via the epidural route (page 116).

EPIDURAL ANALGESIA

Epidural analgesia has probably produced the most beneficial impact on equine analgesia of any technique in the last 5–10 years. It is now routinely used in many equine clinics throughout the world. It can be used both acutely around the time of surgery and also for days or even weeks of treatment via a catheter in horses with serious injury, osteomyelitis and other conditions causing substantial long-term pain. Although there is obviously potential for problems such as infection, reports of case series generally show very low rates of complications.

The epidural route of administration targets specific receptors in the dorsal horn of the spinal cord. This has the advantage that unwanted systemic effects are considerably reduced, much smaller doses of the drug are used, and the effect generally lasts longer, as uptake into the circulation is relatively slow. Preservative-free solutions should be used so that the spinal canal is not damaged; however, sodium metabisulphite 0.1% appears to be safe. Formalin-based solutions should definitely be avoided.

By far the most common route of administration in horses is the caudal block, through the first coccygeal space. The meninges reach the midsacral region in horses, hence use of the lumbosacral space runs the risk of a spinal injection. Any surgery or trauma to the hindlimb and perineal region may benefit from epidural analgesia.

Local anaesthetic agents such as lidocaine, mepivacaine, or, for a longer effect, bupivacaine, can be used to supply epidural analgesia in horses. These drugs produce local anaesthesia, hence it is essential that an appropriate volume is used or the hindlimbs are paralysed. Volume is more important than dose, and 7–8 mL of a 2% lidocaine solution is sufficient to block the perineal region of a 500 kg horse. This method gives only 1–2 hours' anaesthesia (3–4 hours with bupivacaine or ropivacaine) and is more commonly used for perineal surgery rather than simply for analgesia. Block takes 15 minutes to develop. Local anaesthetics cannot be used to supply hindlimb analgesia in the standing horse, as the animal will become ataxic or recumbent.

Drugs used for epidural analgesia include opioids, generally morphine, the α_2 agonists, usually detomidine, and occasionally ketamine. Morphine at 0.05–0.1 mg/kg provides up to 24 hours' pain relief for hindlimbs, rear abdomen and the perineal region. It does not affect the nerve conduction responsible for skeletal muscle motor control. Onset of analgesia may take several hours. Very rarely morphine may cause intense pruritus, necessitating appropriate sedation (with acepromazine and systemic α_2 agonists) until the effect has abated, to prevent self-inflicted trauma.

Detomidine, up to 0.03 mg/kg, has become well used by the epidural route and has a more rapid onset than morphine. Its analgesic effect lasts much longer via this route, and although there is an initial systemic effect and sedation, this does not last as long as the analgesia and can be reversed with systemic atipamezole whilst leaving the analgesic effect intact. It is also common practice to use morphine and detomidine together for a synergistic effect. Both are usually given together in a single injection of around 10 mL, to encourage cranial spread. This method has produced good analgesia and is probably the most routine combination now used clinically.

Xylazine can be used by the epidural route, but because it has some local anaesthetic effects is likely to cause hindlimb ataxia. Hence, in horses detomidine is the preferred α_2 agonist for epidural administration.

Ketamine (0.5–1.0 mg/kg) has been used, although there is only limited clinical experience with this drug. There is some concern that the low pH of ketamine solutions may cause spinal damage, but this has not occurred in the research horses treated in this way.

Epidural analgesia is used most commonly for perioperative analgesia, usually as a single injection of morphine or morphine plus detomidine. It is most logical to give this before induction of anaesthesia, to gain all the benefits of pre-emptive analgesia. This is most appropriate for hindlimb surgery, particularly if bilateral. It may also be appropriate for laparotomy. It is advantageous for standing laparoscopy, as the epidural route produces fair analgesia of the peritoneum.

A second common use for epidural analgesia is during treatment of chronic, debilitating hindlimb lameness. Infected tendon sheaths, joints and the like may cause very severe pain for some weeks during treatment. Epidural analgesia, preferably via a catheter rather than repeated injections, makes a substantial contribution to the wellbeing of the horse and its response to treatment. Morphine, or morphine and detomidine, can be injected two to three times daily.

Technique

Strict aseptic precautions are essential, and it is worth using a proper spinal needle with a short bevel and stylet rather than a regular hypodermic needle. Disposable spinal needles are commercially available in a wide range of sizes, suitable even for the very large horse. These needles give a better 'feel', making placement more certain. The site over the first coccygeal space is clipped and scrubbed for surgery. The site is located as a depression behind the midline prominence (C1) immediately behind a line drawn between the two points of the hip (Figure 6.5). Pumping the tail may help to locate the site. Local anaesthetic solution is placed intradermally over the site and then

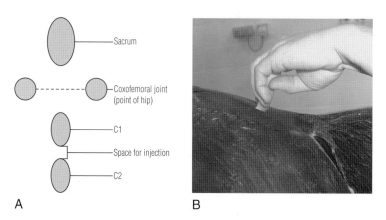

FIG 6.5 (A) Location of the site for caudal epidural injection. (B) The first coccygeal space is palpated as a depression in the midline. If the sacrococcygeal space can be palpated it is also suitable for epidural injection.

down towards the spine. A spinal needle (20G, 6–10 cm) is then inserted in the midline at right-angles to the skin in both planes (Figure 6.6a). A popping sensation may be appreciated as the needle goes through the ligamentum flavum. The needle is pushed on in until it hits bone and is then withdrawn slightly. The stylet is removed, and if the needle is positioned correctly, hissing of air into the negative pressure epidural space may be heard. Alternatively, if the correct site has been located a drop of saline placed on the end of the needle will be sucked in. A further test is to inject air, which will go without resistance or compression (Figure 6.6b). Attempts are made to reposition the needle if the space has not been entered. Injection should be slow and steady.

Longer-term analgesia can best be provided by placing an epidural catheter. This is rarely required for surgical analgesia alone, but may be of considerable benefit afterwards and for the care of horses with chronic severe hindlimb pain.

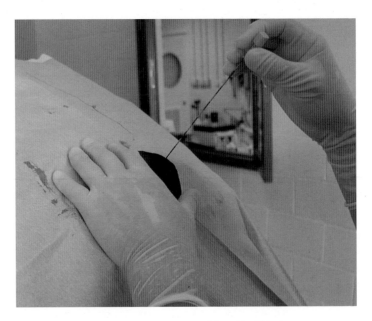

FIG 6.6a Epidural injection. A spinal needle is used for epidural injection.

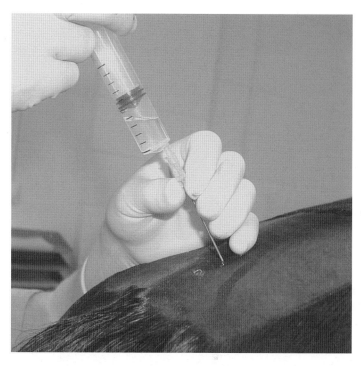

FIG 6.6b *The air test confirms the correct placement of the needle in the epidural space. The solution is injected easily without compression of air in the syringe.*

An epidural catheter is placed under very stringent aseptic conditions. Disposable epidural packs (e.g. Mila) are available, with appropriate equipment for use in horses. A Tuohy needle is placed in the same way as the spinal needle for the simple injection. The Tuohy needle has a forward-facing curved bevel, which allows the catheter to be passed through the needle and forwards up the epidural space once the needle has been correctly placed (Figure 6.7a). The catheter should be threaded in at least 4–6 cm, or more if a more cranial effect is required. It is then secured securely and aseptically to the skin and covered with an adhesive dressing; a bacterial filter should be included at the injection port, and all handling and injection must be strictly aseptic (Figure 6.7b).

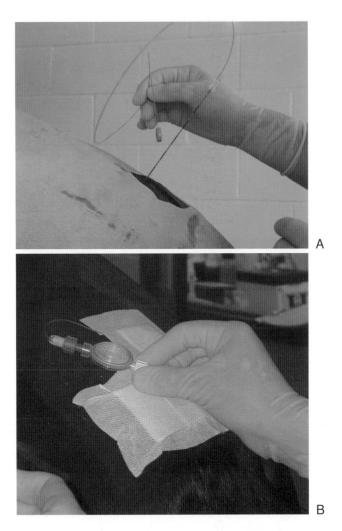

FIG 6.7 Epidural catheter. (A) The catheter is threaded up the epidural space through the Tuohy needle. (B) Handling and injection using the epidural catheter must be strictly aseptic.

PERIOPERATIVE ANALGESIA

All the above agents and techniques may be used to provide perioperative analgesia. Premedication with NSAIDs and opioids is relatively common practice, although the controversy over perioperative opioid use is still unresolved. α_2-agonists and ketamine are routinely used for their sedative and anaesthetic effects, and may be providing more pre-emptive analgesia than we realise. Postoperative NSAIDs, and less commonly opioids, are also well-established treatments. IV infusion of lidocaine or ketamine, as well as epidural administration of opioids and α_2 agonists, are now well established in equine practice. Long-term pain relief with systemic infusion of opioids, α_2 agonists, ketamine, or combinations of these and other groups of drugs has still to be fully evaluated in horses. Treatment of chronic pain is not the issue in horses as in small animal pets, but long-term use of NSAIDs to keep older horses active in sport and recreation has worked well in the past and has yet to be superseded by newer techniques.

Further reading

Bennett RC and Steffey EP (2002) Use of opioids for pain and anaesthetic management in horses. *Veterinary Clinics of North America. Equine Practice* **18**: 47–60.

Brianceau P, Chevalier H, Karas A, et al (2002) Intravenous lidocaine and small intestinal size, abdominal fluid, and outcome after colic surgery in horses. *Journal of Veterinary Internal Medicine* **16**: 763–741.

Burford JH and Cortey KT (2006) Morphine-associated pruritis after single extradural administration in a horse. *Veterinary Anaesthesia & Analgesia* **33**: 193–198.

Goodrich LR, Nixon AJ, Fubini SL, et al (2002) Epidural morphine and detomidine decreases postoperative hindlimb lameness in horses after bilateral stifle arthroscopy. *Veterinary Surgery* **31**: 232–239.

Hall LW and Clarke KW (1991) *Veterinary Anaesthesia*, 9th edn. Baillière Tindall, London, 80–95, 217–220.

Martin CA, Kerr CL, Pearce SG, et al (2003) Outcome of epidural catheterisation for delivery of analgesics in horses: 43 cases (1998–2001). *Journal of the American Veterinary Medical Association* **222**: 1394–1398.

Matthews NS, Fielding CI and Swinebroad E (2004) How to use a ketamine constant rate infusion in horses for analgesia. Proceedings of the 50th Annual Convention of the AAEP, 1431.

Mircica E, Clutton RE, Kyles KW, et al (2003) Problems associated with perioperative morphine in horses: a retrospective case analysis. *Veterinary Anaesthesia and Analgesia* **30**: 147–155.

Price J, Catriona S, Welsh EM, et al (2003) Preliminary evaluation of a behaviour-based system for assessment of postoperative pain in horses following arthroscopic surgery. *Veterinary Anaesthesia and Analgesia* **30**: 123–137.

Senior JM, Pinchbeck GL, Dugdale AH, et al (2004) Retrospective study of the risk factors and prevalence of colic in horses after orthopaedic surgery. *Veterinary Record* **155**: 321–325.

Taylor PM, Pascoe PJ and Mama K (2002) Diagnosing and treating pain in the horse – where are we today? *Veterinary Clinics of North America. Equine Practice* **18**: 1–19.

Thomasy SM, Slovis N, Maxwell LK, et al (2004) Transdermal fentanyl combined with nonsteroidal anti-inflammatory drugs for analgesia in horses. *Journal of Veterinary Internal Medicine* **18**: 550–554.

7

ANAESTHETIC PROBLEMS

The risk of death during or associated with general anaesthesia is much higher in horses than in other domestic species or humans. The reasons for this are not entirely clear, but some of the problems that may arise are described here. It is important to realise that even when anaesthesia is apparently uneventful, postoperative problems may occur.

INDUCTION

In virtually all cases anaesthesia is induced when the horse is standing; in the course of becoming unconscious it must also lie down. Injury to both horse and handler may occur at this stage, particularly if the horse becomes excited or ataxic. If the horse already has an injury, such as a fractured limb, this may become irreparably damaged by an uncontrolled induction. There are numerous approaches for smoothing the transition to unconsciousness in the horse.

SEDATION/INDUCTION AGENTS
Appropriate sedation is the mainstay of a smooth induction. This ranges from minimal tranquillisation, such as calming a nervous horse with acepromazine, to deep sedation with α_2 agonists and opioids that allows mechanical support to be used. A quiet environment is essential in all cases and worth making considerable effort to achieve.

FREE-STANDING
Intravenous induction of anaesthesia with the horse standing unsupported is a common technique (Figure 7.1). For the horse, this is most safely carried out in a padded recovery box, as even if it becomes ataxic or excited the risk of new injury is fairly low. This technique is less well suited to a horse with a fractured limb, as it may become very ataxic standing on three legs. Techniques using smaller doses of α_2 agonists should be used where ataxia is likely to be a particular problem. Free-standing inductions are also appropriate in a large space such as a field or barn, where there is nothing for the horse to run into. This is also safer for handlers, who have space to get out of the way of the horse if necessary. Free-standing inductions are not advisable in restricted surroundings with projections such as mangers and water troughs. The horse should be discouraged from moving about between administration

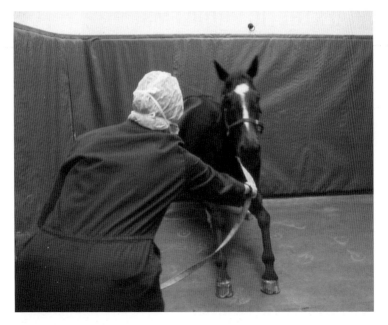

FIG 7.1 A free-standing induction in a padded recovery box is commonly used for routine major and minor surgery.

of heavy premedication and induction, as this may lead to marked ataxia and excitement. Better control is provided by head and tail ropes to prevent the horse from swinging around. This depends on availability of suitably placed, strong ring attachments (Figure 7.2).

SUPPORT FROM HANDLERS

This is the simplest approach to a controlled induction and requires the least specialist equipment. With a little attention to detail this is a highly effective means of helping a horse to slide smoothly into lateral recumbency. It is best done against a smooth, solid wall that is at least slightly longer than the horse from head to tail. Ideally the wall should be padded, but it must be non-abrasive. Brick or concrete is not suitable. This technique is well suited to use in a padded recovery box where there are no other means of support (Figure 7.3).

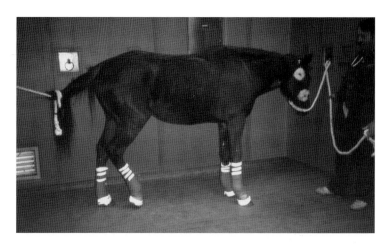

FIG 7.2   Greater control at induction is achieved with head and tail ropes. Safely secured wall rings which are at least as high as the horse's head are essential.

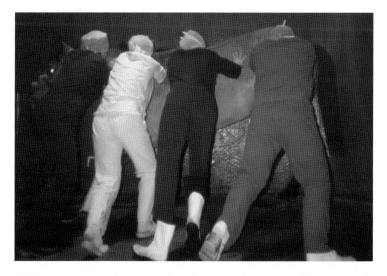

FIG 7.3   Good control at induction can be achieved when there is no specialist equipment by using at least four people to push the horse against a smooth, solid wall as anaesthesia is induced.

At least half of the handlers should be experienced. The horse is held parallel to the wall and as close as possible to it. One handler should hold the head with a headcollar and rope, and the rest should be spaced out ready to lean on the horse and keep it upright as it sinks into sternal recumbency. The number of handlers depends on the size of the horse, but there should be at least one at the shoulder and one at the hindquarters. If the horse has a fractured limb a further individual should be designated to support and protect the limb as the horse goes down.

The same approach can be used in a large space with an equal number of people on either side of the horse. It is essential that there is room for handlers to get out of the way of the horse if induction is not as smooth as anticipated. Both techniques depend on a smooth, slow induction. Techniques based on α_2 agonists, ketamine, opioids, acepromazine and diazepam as well as guaiphenesin/barbiturate have all been used in this way. Calm, quiet handling of the horse is essential.

SQUEEZE BOX OR SWINGING DOOR

This technique is the most easily perfected, particularly when only a few people, or only inexperienced helpers, are available. It usually requires a purpose-built door or gate; this is a relatively simple matter if a recovery box is being constructed and is a great deal more simple than a tilt table (Figure 7.4a&b).

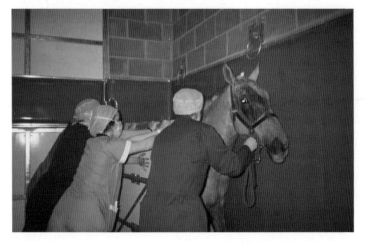

FIG 7.4a The most practical additional equipment for controlling induction is the squeeze box.

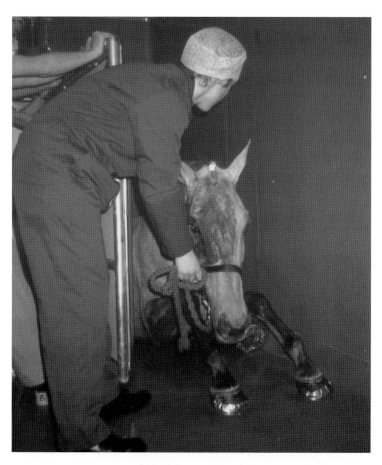

FIG 7.4b Induction is safely controlled by a few people applying pressure to the door as the horse becomes recumbent.

The horse is positioned behind the door with its hindquarters up against the hinged wall, and the door is closed on to it. As anaesthesia is induced the door is pushed against the horse to support it in an upright position as it sinks into sternal recumbency. It is possible to achieve the same effect as the handler technique described above, but with fewer people and considerably less risk of injury to personnel.

THE TILT TABLE

A tilt table is an extremely effective way of moving the horse smoothly from standing to lateral recumbency (Figure 7.5). It does, however, require complex equipment and experienced handlers. A mismanaged tilt-table induction is more dangerous than any free-standing induction. Success with this

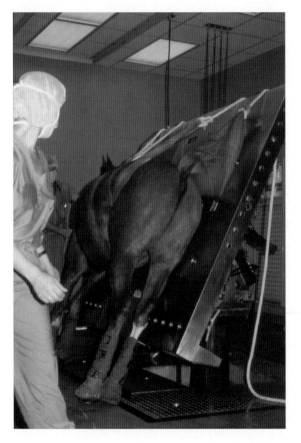

FIG 7.5 A tilt table provides maximum control at induction but requires complex equipment and experienced personnel.

technique depends on appropriate induction to ensure that the horse is relaxed but not too ataxic, and then swift, calm operation of belly bands and tilt controls as unconsciousness develops. It should not be attempted without several people familiar with the process.

SLINGS, BELLY BANDS

There are a number of other techniques adapted by some clinics to enhance induction. Slings designed for helicopter horse-rescue can be very effectively used at induction, especially if the horse has become accustomed to their use beforehand (Figure 7.6). In this case anaesthesia is induced with the horse standing in the slings and once it has lost consciousness it is slowly lowered to the floor or on to a means of transport. This is particularly valuable for horses with a major limb fracture, especially as slings may be an important component of pre- and postoperative treatment. Again, the technique requires at least some of the handlers to be experienced.

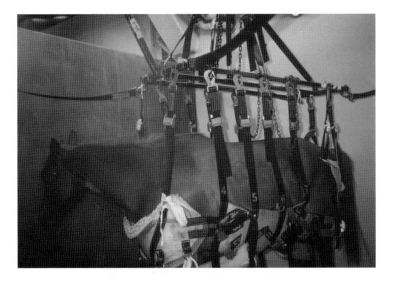

FIG 7.6 Induction of anaesthesia in slings is greatly facilitated if the horse has already become accustomed to this form of support. Such preoperative preparation is particularly worthwhile if the horse is also likely to require slings after surgery.

MAINTENANCE

Most serious problems occur during maintenance of anaesthesia, although the effects may not be manifest until the horse begins to regain consciousness. As a rule, general anaesthesia depresses many systems in the body. Obviously the CNS is depressed, in order to produce anaesthesia, but other systems are also affected by most anaesthetic agents.

HYPOTENSION

All volatile anaesthetics cause hypotension. The effect is particularly notorious in the horse, and is probably one of the major causes of the high anaesthetic risk in this species. Hypotension results from myocardial depression and peripheral vasodilation. Myocardial depression is particularly marked with halothane, but is not insignificant with isoflurane and sevoflurane. It leads to a fall in cardiac output and poor tissue perfusion. There is a strong association between hypotension during anaesthesia and development of postoperative myopathy, which is discussed in detail below. The more subtle effects of poor perfusion are not well understood, but low cardiac output may be one of the most serious side effects of general anaesthesia in horses.

It is virtually impossible to assess arterial blood pressure without measuring it. Pulse quality relates to the difference between diastolic and systolic pressure. Although the pulse is usually stronger at higher pressures this is not always the case; pulse quality cannot be used to measure blood pressure. Fortunately it is a relatively simple matter to measure arterial blood pressure in horses and this should be routine, at least where volatile agents are used (pages 89–94).

Treatment
It is common practice to support blood pressure during volatile-agent anaesthesia and there is good circumstantial evidence that this reduces the risk of postoperative myopathy; it should be considered good clinical practice. Both blood pressure (driving pressure) and cardiac output (flow) are important. Cardiac output and blood pressure are directly related:

$$\text{blood pressure} = \text{cardiac output} \times \text{peripheral resistance.}$$

However, because it is easy to measure arterial blood pressure and difficult to measure cardiac output, the clinical approach is to increase blood pressure using methods that increase cardiac output. Three approaches can be combined to ensure mean arterial blood pressure is kept above 70 mmHg. These depend first on reducing the amount of volatile anaesthetic delivered by using supplementary IV agents (pages 77–79); second, on fluid infusion to prevent hypovolaemia and ensure adequate venous return; and third, on the use of inotropes to support cardiac contractility (pages 80–81).

CARDIAC DYSRHYTHMIAS

Bradycardia

Bradycardia is not uncommon in anaesthetised horses and may cause low cardiac output and hypotension. Very slow sinus rhythm (fewer than 20 beats per min, bpm) is sometimes seen in fit, racing Thoroughbreds; the long periods between beats increase the potential for ventricular fibrillation. Second-degree atrioventricular (AV) block is not uncommon, especially when α_2 agonist sedatives have been given, and may also cause a low ventricular rate. Most of these bradydysrhythmias are caused by high vagal tone and respond to anticholinergic treatment. A heart rate less than 25 bpm should be treated with anticholinergics.

Glycopyrrolate (0.005–0.01 mg/kg – slow IV) has little CNS effect and usually increases heart rate steadily, without dysrhythmias. If inotrope infusion is in progress a transient but spectacular tachycardia may develop. Glycopyrrolate should be given before inotrope infusion begins if possible. The effect of glycopyrrolate may wane after 1–2 hours and a second (smaller) dose may be required.

Atropine (0.005–0.02 mg/kg) may briefly exacerbate the bradycardia through a central effect. The same tachycardia is seen if inotropes are being infused. Atropine appears to be longer acting than glycopyrrolate in horses, and any effect decreasing gut motility may last longer.

Hyoscine (0.1 mg/kg) is also successful. This conservative dose may need repeating after 15–30 minutes.

Atrial fibrillation

Atrial fibrillation occasionally develops during anaesthesia. This may have little effect on blood pressure if the ventricular rate remains normal. However, it is not uncommon for blood pressure to fall, because ventricular filling is decreased. It is usually sufficient to increase venous return by electrolyte infusion; one or more additional wide-lumen IV catheters should be placed as soon as possible to allow this. The inspired volatile agent should be reduced as much as possible and a normal heart rate should be the aim. Anticholinergics should not be given as this may increase ventricular rate to the atrial rate, drastically reducing stroke volume and cardiac output. A slow heart rate allows time for the ventricles to fill and maintains cardiac output. It is probably better to avoid drugs that might affect heart rhythm, such as sympathomimetics or α_2 agonists. However, dobutamine has been used to increase blood pressure in horses with atrial fibrillation and is the agent of choice if increasing fluid infusion does not resolve hypotension.

Ideally, horses found to be in atrial fibrillation before elective surgery should be treated to convert to sinus rhythm before anaesthesia. This is possible with quinidine, but electrical cardioversion requires anaesthesia for the treatment. The approach to anaesthesia outlined above is employed. In such cases, acepromazine and opioids are best used for premedication; if α_2 agonists are required low doses should be used. Guaiphenesin and barbiturates or ketamine have been used for induction, and isoflurane or sevoflurane should be chosen for maintenance rather than halothane.

Ventricular dysrhythmias

Ventricular dysrhythmias do not commonly develop during anaesthesia in non-toxic horses. However, volatile agents, particularly halothane, sensitise the heart to catecholamine-induced dysrhythmias and premature ventricular ectopic contractions may occasionally be seen. Individual ectopic beats that do not seriously affect cardiac output do not themselves need treating. Nevertheless, they may indicate some systemic disorder and causes such as hypoxaemia, hypercapnia, electrolyte abnormalities or excessive sympathetic stimulation should be sought and treated. If halothane is in use it should be changed to isoflurane or sevoflurane if available. Ventricular dysrhythmias are also occasionally seen in response to IV injection of potentiated sulphonamides and surgical use of catecholamines. In these cases repeat doses must not be given and the effect usually wears off without further treatment.

Ventricular dysrhythmias that are increasing in frequency and affecting output should be treated with lidocaine (0.5 mg/kg). A single dose is given first; this can be repeated if necessary, up to a total of 0.2 mg/kg. Infusion is rarely required during anaesthesia in horses if the underlying cause is successfully identified and treated.

The ultimate arrhythmia is cardiac arrest, which is discussed under resuscitation (pages 171–174).

HYPOXAEMIA

In horses, anaesthesia and recumbency cause hypoxaemia, which may be seen even when high oxygen concentrations are inspired. In the standing horse there is little difference between alveolar and arterial oxygen tensions. However, in the anaesthetised horse the arterial oxygen tension may be very much lower than in the alveoli. This occurs in laterally or dorsally recumbent horses because the lower lung fields are compressed by the weight of abdominal viscera pressing through the dome-shaped diaphragm (Figure 7.7). The problem is usually worst in larger horses lying in dorsal recumbency. Blood flowing through the compressed lungs does not become fully oxygenated because the compressed lung is poorly ventilated. This may result from actual 'shunt', where the blood does not come into contact with any ventilated alveoli, or from ventilation–perfusion (V/Q) mismatch, where ventilation of an area is inadequate for maximum oxygenation but not completely absent. The poorly oxygenated blood joins any coming from well-ventilated areas and

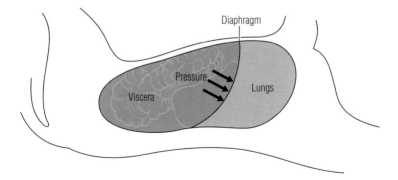

FIG 7.7 Diagram of horse in dorsal recumbency. The dependent lung fields are compressed, so that although they are perfused, ventilation is reduced or absent. This leads to venous admixture in the pulmonary veins and results in arterial hypoxaemia.

lowers the final arterial oxygen tension in the blood leaving the lung in the pulmonary veins. Centrally induced respiratory depression will enhance hypoxaemia, but if the horse is breathing a high inspired oxygen fraction the major cause of hypoxaemia is the compressed lung.

Low arterial oxygen tension may limit oxygen delivery to the tissues and is potentially harmful. The anaesthetised horse is likely to become hypoxaemic unless high inspired oxygen concentrations are supplied; even when breathing 100% oxygen some horses are relatively hypoxaemic. It is almost impossible to assess arterial oxygenation without some means of measurement. Pulse oximetry measures haemoglobin oxygen saturation and blood gas analysis measures the tension or pressure of the gas, and at least one of these should be used if available (Chapter 5).

Prevention/treatment
No measures are entirely effective and their importance in improving outcome has not been conclusively tested.

A high inspired oxygen fraction. In most cases during volatile agent anaesthesia oxygen is used as the carrier gas and the inspired oxygen fraction will be close to 100%. However, if nitrous oxide has been given, or low flows were used and nitrogen has not cleared from the lungs, it may be possible to increase the inspired oxygen a little further by eliminating the other gases from the circuit. Hypoxaemia is not uncommon in larger horses even when 100% is inspired. In human anaesthesia high inspired oxygen concentrations are associated with poorer oxygenation as a result of alveolar collapse when all the oxygen is absorbed. As a consequence, oxygenated air is often used as the carrier gas because nitrogen is considered the skeleton of the lung, keeping the alveoli open. This may be applicable to some horses but has not yet been evaluated.

Reduce the pressure from the abdominal content. Preoperative starvation reduces the gut content and increases the functional residual capacity of the lung. This may help oxygenation but the beneficial effect is limited, as it impossible to empty the gut completely. Starvation should not exceed 12–18 hours or the horse will be more agitated and metabolic changes develop.

Mechanical ventilation. Intermittent positive-pressure ventilation, IPPV, may improve oxygenation slightly but tends to increase ventilation to areas already adequately expanded without re-expanding the compressed sections.

Improve the ventilation–perfusion mismatch. This would be an ideal mechanism to improve oxygenation, but there is no easy solution. Preferential ventilation of lower lung fields is not yet a viable clinical technique, and application of positive end-expiratory pressure (PEEP) depresses cardiac output. Pharmacological methods are equally controversial. Clenbuterol (0.4–0.8 mg/kg) is a β_2 adrenoceptor agonist that has been shown to increase the arterial oxygen tension. The results are variable, the side effects of tachycardia and sweating marked, and the clinical benefits unproven. Aerosolised salbutamol (albuterol) (2 µg/kg, for example 10 'puffs' of human commercial preparations supplying 100 µg per 'puff') given via the endotracheal tube has also been shown to increase arterial oxygen tension and has less systemic effect than clenbuterol. Arterial oxygenation generally improves considerably, but in some horses the effect is limited. However, the effect of either clenbuterol or aerosolised salbutamol on actual oxygen delivery is not clear.

Change the horse's position. Hypoxaemia is worse in dorsal than lateral recumbency, and moving a horse from dorsal to lateral may improve oxygenation. However, this is rarely practical during surgery. If there is a choice between dorsal or lateral recumbency for a particular procedure, lateral is preferable. Occasionally it is possible to improve oxygenation by tilting the table so that the horse's head is higher than the abdomen, to take some weight off the diaphragm. However, this often has minimal effect and may cause undesirable alterations in peripheral circulation. The practical problems of holding the horse at a considerable angle usually negate any benefit.

Increase oxygen delivery. Although insufficient oxygen supply to the tissues must be potentially deleterious it is difficult to assess how serious the hypoxaemia is at a practical clinical level. Arterial oxygenation is only part of the equation: cardiac output and oxygen delivery are what matters; it is probable that depression of cardiac output and hypotension are more important than the precise blood oxygen content in ensuring oxygen delivery in anaesthetised horses. Measures to increase cardiac output (pages 80–81) are probably the most practical and effective way to improve oxygen supply to the tissues.

SPECIAL NEEDS OF THE HORSE WITH CHRONIC OBSTRUCTIVE PULMONARY DISEASE (COPD)

In this condition the small airways of the lungs are constricted with secretions and high smooth muscle tone. As a result of ventilation–perfusion mismatch, resting arterial oxygen tension is lower than normal. The degree of hypoxaemia is rarely life-threatening. A slight increase in respiratory drive usually occurs, and arterial carbon dioxide tension is usually normal or slightly low. For elective surgery, management in dust-free conditions and a course of bronchodilator therapy usually renders such horses symptom free and anaesthesia may proceed as normal. Horses with symptoms of COPD may require anaesthesia in emergency or where management was not completely successful. Although this disease must presumably increase the anaesthetic risk, in practice most horses with COPD are not more difficult to anaesthetise. The increased respiratory drive from mild hypoxaemia persists in anaesthesia and respiratory depression is less marked than usual. In addition, most volatile agents used in horses reduce bronchial tone and improve the condition. All the methods described above may be used to manage hypoxaemia. Occasionally, a high respiratory rate is seen, in which case respiration may be inefficient as expiratory time is inadequate for gas conduction through constricted airways. In this case it is better to use IPPV at a slow rate with a larger tidal volume.

HYPERCAPNIA

General anaesthesia in horses almost invariably leads to central respiratory depression and carbon dioxide retention. This may be exacerbated by hyperoxia from breathing a high inspired oxygen fraction. Hypercapnia leads to respiratory acidosis, which increases sympathetic stimulation and may, at least theoretically, increase the chance of cardiac dysrhythmias in the presence of volatile anaesthetic agents. However, the degree of acidosis common during equine anaesthesia rarely appears to cause a clinical problem. The sympathetic stimulation induced by carbon dioxide tensions up to around 80 mmHg (10.7 kPa) actually improves cardiac output and blood pressure; this is probably beneficial.

It is impossible to assess arterial carbon dioxide tension without some means of measurement. Anaesthetised horses rarely increase respiration in response to hypercapnia, since CNS depression is the underlying cause of the carbon dioxide retention. End-tidal (approximately alveolar) carbon dioxide measurement gives a guide to arterial carbon dioxide but may under estimate by 10–20 mmHg (1–3 kPa) (pages 97–99). Blood gas analysis is required for accurate information (pages 100–101).

Prevention/treatment

It is generally accepted that hypercapnia above approximately 75 mmHg (10 kPa) should be treated. A more logical approach may be to base the decision to treat on the degree of acidosis. If possible, the pH should not fall below 7.20.

Reduce the CNS depression. Respiratory depression is a result of anaesthetic-induced depression of the respiratory centre, hence reducing the depth of anaesthesia may improve ventilation. In horses, surgical anaesthesia can rarely be achieved without a certain degree of respiratory depression. As the animal no longer responds to hypercapnia, low oxygen becomes the stimulus to breathe and high arterial oxygen may depress respiration further.

Ventilation. Carbon dioxide retention is easily treated by increasing ventilation. Even with large areas of compressed lung, increased ventilation of the rest will lower the arterial carbon dioxide tension. This is most effectively achieved with mechanical ventilation, although assisted ventilation by manual compression of the rebreathing bag is feasible, if laborious.

POSTOPERATIVE MYOPATHY

Postoperative myopathy causes serious postanaesthetic morbidity in horses. Although signs are first seen in the recovery period the damage has occurred during anaesthesia.

Clinical signs

Postoperative myopathy is seen most commonly in large, well-muscled horses, particularly after prolonged periods of general anaesthesia. It is usually evident as soon as the horse tries to stand, but occasionally signs may not develop for a few hours. The muscle groups affected are generally those that were dependent during anaesthesia, usually the triceps after lateral recumbency and the gluteals after dorsal recumbency. Occasionally, non-dependent limbs are affected. The problem is seen less commonly in lighter animals and after short periods of anaesthesia. Clinical signs range from mild lameness to severe generalised myopathy, where the horse cannot stand. The affected muscles are hard, swollen and painful. Undoubtedly some cases of so-called postoperative radial paralysis are in fact myopathy; it may be difficult to distinguish between myopathy and neuropathy because nerve and muscle may both be affected by the same process. Myopathy is striking in the degree of pain that it causes (Figure 7.8). Affected animals are extremely distressed and may be difficult to manage. They sweat copiously, breathing is laboured and rapid, and the horse tends to be very restless. When the hindlimbs are

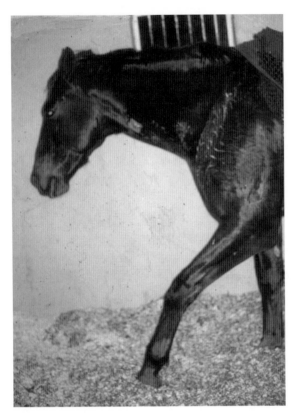

FIG 7.8 *Postoperative myopathy causes marked pain. This horse has myopathy in the left triceps. It is unable to bear weight on the left forelimb, the muscle is hard and swollen and the horse is sweating, distressed to the point of hyperventilating, and restless – all cardinal signs of severe pain.*

affected the horse may be unable to position itself for urination, thereby adding to its discomfort.

Serum creatine kinase (CK) and aspartate aminotransferase (AST) activity is increased, but may not correlate with the degree of lameness. High CK values recorded within a few hours of the end of anaesthesia confirm the diagnosis, but normal or only slightly raised values do not necessarily exclude it. Myoglobin released into the circulation from damaged muscle leads to the production of dark red or brown urine. Large quantities of myoglobin may block and damage the kidney tubules, causing pain or even fatal renal failure. When the horse begins to move or stands up, there is a transient increase in blood lactate from reperfusion of areas compressed during recumbency.

Pathogenesis

Postoperative myopathy appears to result from ischaemic damage to muscles that were underperfused during anaesthesia. A combination of volatile agent-induced hypotension, pressure on compressed muscle groups and restricted venous drainage is responsible. Time is a significant factor: muscles that are ischaemic for long periods are more likely to be affected. The aetiology of rare generalised myopathy or malignant hyperthermia is less clear, but may also be triggered by underperfusion. Glycogen storage disease (page 205) may also predispose to the development of postoperative myopathy.

Hypotension. It is now widely accepted that intraoperative hypotension leads to postoperative myopathy since this was convincingly demonstrated by two studies from North America. Strong empirical evidence from more recent clinical equine anaesthetic practice indicates that the incidence of severe myopathy is much reduced when efforts are made to maintain mean arterial blood pressure above approximately 70 mmHg.

Intracompartmental pressure. Postoperative myopathy in horses has many features in common with the compartmental syndrome in humans, where decreased muscle perfusion causes severe myopathy. The syndrome is seen after trauma where the muscle swells, and in athletes with well-developed muscle bodies. The syndrome can occur in any group of muscles that are contained within an inextensible envelope (a compartment) usually made up of muscle fascia and adjacent periosteum (Figure 7.9). Such a compartment has no outlet for the relief of applied pressure and can expand very little in volume; the consequence is an increase in pressure within. In the compartmental syndrome a cycle of events is set up in which pressure in the compartment rises, due either to external pressure or to trauma-induced damage causing cellular swelling. Increased pressure prevents capillary perfusion and causes ischaemia, ischaemia causes hypoxia, hypoxia causes further cell damage and swelling, swelling increases the pressure, and the cycle is set up (Figure 7.10).

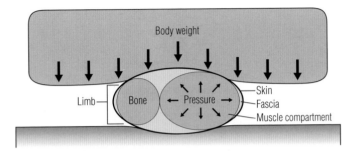

Operating table

FIG 7.9 An osteofascial compartment that cannot expand in volume is prone to development of compartmental syndrome if the pressure within the compartment rises. On the operating table, the horse's body weight pressing on dependent limb muscles causes the pressure in such osteofascial compartments to increase.

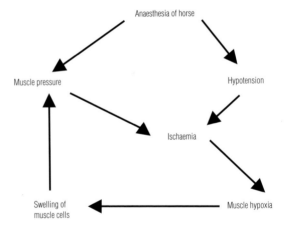

FIG 7.10 Development of the compartmental syndrome depends on a vicious cycle being set up: the horse's body weight on dependent muscle increases the pressure within the compartment. If arterial driving pressure is low, as with the hypotension that occurs during volatile agent anaesthesia, muscle perfusion is inadequate and myocytes become ischaemic. Cells lacking oxygen and building up waste products begin to swell, which further increases the compartment pressure, thereby exacerbating the effect.

This cycle is easily set up in the dependent muscle groups in anaesthetised horses. A number of investigators have measured the compartmental pressures in anaesthetised horses and found them to be high enough to prevent normal perfusion. A driving pressure (mean arterial pressure minus compartment pressure) of 30 mmHg is required to keep capillary blood flowing. Dependent-limb compartment pressures of 35–65 mmHg are not uncommon (normal is less than 10 mmHg). To achieve a driving pressure of 30 mmHg, mean arterial pressures of at least 65 and often up to 95 mmHg are required (Figure 7.11). Horses anaesthetised with volatile agents are often more hypotensive than this. It is not surprising that anaesthetised horses suffer from muscle ischaemia.

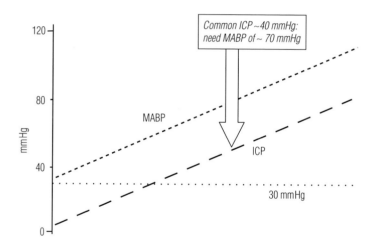

FIG 7.11 The relationship between mean arterial blood pressure (MABP) and compartmental pressure (ICP). A driving pressure of 30 mmHg is required between MABP and ICP to ensure muscle perfusion. A minimum of 30 mmHg MABP (....................) is required at normal ICP pressures. As ICP rises (– – – – – –), MABP (- - - - - -) needs to remain 30 mmHg above in order to maintain perfusion. ICPs of 35–45 mmHg are common in anaesthetised horses, hence a MABP goal of 70 mmHg or above is logical.

Venous drainage. Obstructed venous drainage stops blood flow and is equally effective in preventing adequate muscle perfusion. Limbs held in abnormal positions may have obstructed venous outflow, which will exacerbate any perfusion deficiencies in the equine limb during anaesthesia. In horses in lateral recumbency, drawing the non-dependent forelimb back hard to allow access to medial structures on the dependent limb appears to obstruct venous drainage from the upper limb and probably causes upper limb triceps myopathy (Figure 7.12).

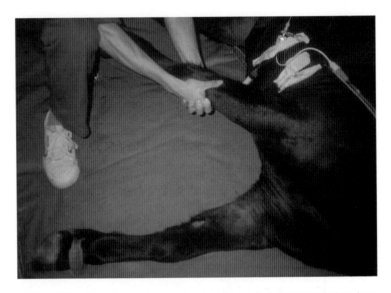

FIG 7.12 *Pulling the non-dependent forelimb back hard in the laterally recumbent horse reduces venous drainage from that limb and may cause postoperative myopathy.*

Hypoxaemia. Poor oxygen supply to the muscle undoubtedly contributes to muscle hypoxia, hence low arterial oxygen tension presumably increases the likelihood of myopathy. However, it appears that perfusion is infinitely more important: the tissues extract oxygen efficiently as long as there is flowing blood to extract it from.

Prevention

Adequate perfusion in skeletal muscle should prevent postoperative myopathy. This may be achieved by preventing hypotension and poor peripheral perfusion and by careful positioning, both to minimise pressure on dependent muscles and not to restrict venous outflow.

Prevent hypotension. This depends on the three approaches outlined previously (pages 77–81): less volatile agent, fluid infusion, and inotropes. It is generally accepted that mean arterial blood pressure should be maintained at at least 70 mmHg. Although this does not ensure perfusion pressures of 30 mmHg in all cases, it is likely to be adequate in most, as long as positioning is good.

Position of the horse. The horse should be placed on the operating table in a position that does not put any part of its body under strain. A leg pulled hard into an abnormal anatomical relation with the rest of the body is liable to have venous outflow restricted and pressure within muscle bellies may be increased. Limbs should be allowed to settle naturally and be secured without force. When the horse is lying in lateral recumbency both non-dependent limbs should be supported parallel with the ground (Figure 7.13), and the dependent forelimb should be pulled forwards to take pressure off the lower triceps (Figure 7.14). If access to the medial side of the dependent forelimb is required it is best to flex the upper limb out of the way (Figure 7.15).

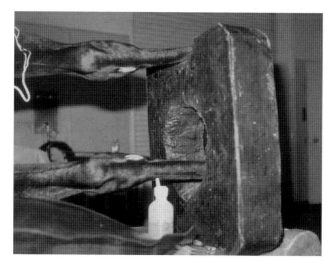

FIG 7.13 In lateral recumbency the horse's legs should be supported parallel to the ground in order to allow maximum venous drainage from the non-dependent limb and to reduce pressure on the dependent limb.

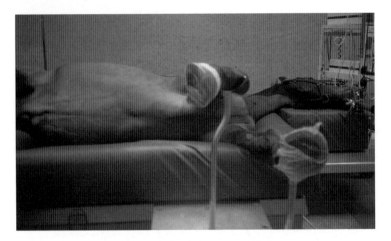

FIG 7.14 *In lateral recumbency the dependent forelimb should be pulled forwards to reduce pressure from the horse's weight on the triceps.*

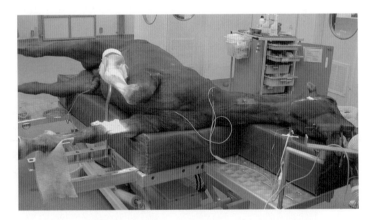

FIG 7.15 *In order to allow access for surgery on the medial side of the dependent forelimb the non-dependent limb should be flexed out of the way and not pulled backwards, as this reduces venous drainage.*

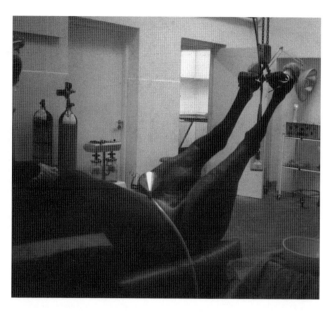

FIG 7.16 It is better to avoid long periods of anaesthesia with both hindlimbs extended as in this illustration. This position increases gluteal muscle pressure. Each leg should be extended separately and the leg not currently undergoing surgery be allowed to relax into a flexed position.

Special precautions are required for the hindlimbs when the horse is in dorsal recumbency. Wide clinical experience has shown that if the hindlimbs are drawn back with the patellae locked (Figure 7.16) the horse may be unable to stand after surgery, although the precise cause is unknown. If this position is absolutely essential for surgery it should be restricted to one limb at a time and as short a period as possible, e.g. 20 minutes. This position should never be used simply to keep the limbs out of the way of the surgery.

Padding the horse. Padding cannot reduce the weight of the horse: all it can do is spread the load over as large an area of the body surface as possible to reduce the pressure at any one site. It is important that the padding is deep enough to prevent the body pressing down on the table at any point or the effect will be lost. Water beds (Figure 7.17) are the most effective, although

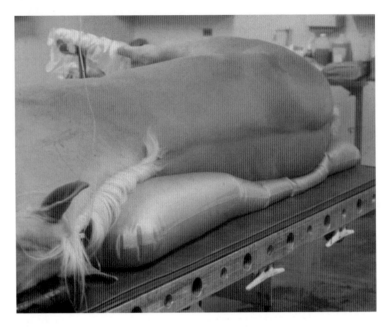

FIG 7.17 Theatre table with waterbed padding. Note that the horse sinks into the bed.

they are cumbersome, expensive, and provide an unstable surgical base. Good results have also been obtained with air mattresses (Figure 7.18) and thick foam sealed in waterproof covers, such as gymnastic mats (Figure 7.19). Air mattresses should not be fully inflated; when fully inflated they are hard and will not support a large area (Figure 7.18).

TREATMENT

If the above procedures were not successful some cases will need treatment. The damage is done during anaesthesia and treatment is largely symptomatic. Reperfusion of ischaemic muscle is probably the point at which the true damage occurs, but this cannot be avoided. It may be possible to prevent the condition worsening by improving perfusion during recovery. In practice, withdrawal of the volatile anaesthetic improves perfusion immediately.

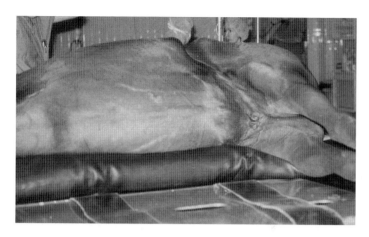

FIG 7.18 Theatre table with air-cushion padding. The cushion is not fully inflated so the horse sinks into the surface. A fully inflated airbed can be almost as hard as concrete!

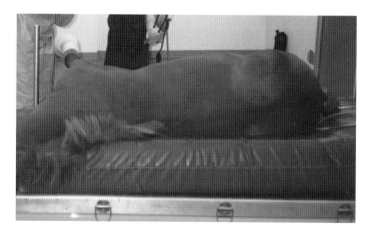

FIG 7.19 Theatre table with covered foam padding.

Analgesia. Pain is often severe and analgesics are an essential part of treatment, both on humanitarian grounds and to make the horse easier to manage.

Non-steroidal anti-inflammatory drugs (NSAIDs). Standard doses of any NSAID are appropriate to this type of injury.

Opioids, e.g. butorphanol (0.02–0.1 mg/kg), morphine (0.1–0.12 mg/kg), methadone (0.1 mg/kg). Potent analgesics may be required, but opioids and NSAIDs can safely be given together.

Sedation. A calm horse is easier to care for, and sedation appears to ease the animal's discomfort. Sedation in combination with opioid analgesia often dramatically alters the horse's demeanour and prevents any opioid-induced box-walking.

Acepromazine (0.03–0.06 mg/kg) is relatively long acting and may improve muscle perfusion; it is an excellent choice for combination with the opioids.

α_2 Agonists. Small doses of xylazine, detomidine or romifidine can help to calm a really distressed horse. They are likely to decrease muscle perfusion and should be used only when analgesia and milder sedation fails to calm the animal adequately.

Diuresis should be instituted in severe cases to prevent myoglobin accumulation in the renal tubules. Large volumes (20–40 L) of intravenous crystalloids should be given. Diuretics are not suitable as they simply dehydrate the horse. If the horse will eat and drink, fluid can be given by mouth. Water can be given by stomach tube if intestinal motility is normal.

Other treatment. Steroids, sodium bicarbonate, dantrolene, diazepam, selenium, vitamin E, dimethyl sulphoxide (DMSO) and ultrasound have all been used with questionable benefit. Ultrasound appears to make the horse more comfortable. Maintaining a horse in slings, if it will tolerate such treatment, may aid recovery in that no further damage is caused (Figure 7.20). The horse should not be forced to keep attempting to stand as it may cause further muscle damage and will undoubtedly become distressed. However, short periods of standing combined with plenty of TLC (tender loving care) will improve the horse's will to live.

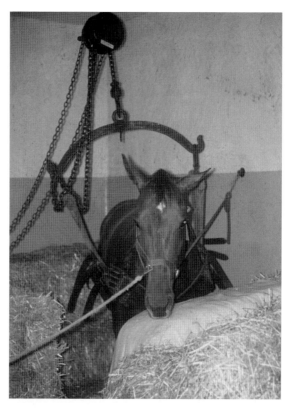

FIG 7.20 Postoperative care of horses with serious fractures or other causes of limited weightbearing is facilitated with slings if the horse will tolerate the support.

NEUROPATHY

Neuropathy is a less common complication of general anaesthesia than myopathy. It may occur under similar conditions as those that cause myopathy, and there is no doubt that some cases of myopathy include an element of neuropathy. Neuropathy itself also occurs as a single entity and, like myopathy, is usually seen as soon as the horse tries to stand after anaesthesia.

Clinical signs

Clinical signs depend on the nerve affected. Radial paralysis is seen (Figure 7.21), and less commonly femoral nerve paralysis may also occur (Figure 7.22). Facial nerve paralysis is not uncommon and is usually seen when the buckle of the headcollar has pressed on the underside of the horse's face (Figure 7.23). Radial or femoral nerve paralysis may be difficult to distinguish from triceps and gluteal myopathy, because pain may prevent the horse from using the affected muscle groups so that the muscles appear paralysed. The two are even more difficult to distinguish in the recumbent horse. The most obvious difference is the absence of pain in the horse with pure neuropathy. The final outcome depends on the extent of the neurological deficit. Laryngeal paralysis may occur in a horse in dorsal recumbency if the neck is overextended and the weight of the head stretches the recurrent laryngeal nerve (see Figure 7.30).

Aetiology

Compressed or hypoxic nerve is susceptible to damage in a similar manner as muscle. It is likely that postoperative neuropathy occurs as a result of ischaemia-induced hypoxia from direct pressure on the nerve or on the arterial supply.

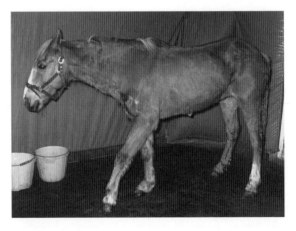

FIG 7.21 The clinical signs of radial paralysis are similar to those of triceps myopathy (see Figure 7.8) but pain is often absent.

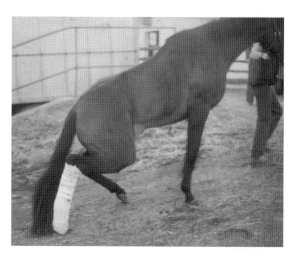

FIG 7.22 *Femoral nerve paralysis results in this characteristic posture of the affected hindlimb with lowered hindquarters. Horses with bilateral femoral nerve paralysis are unable to stand. (Photograph courtesy of Dr L Klein.)*

Obstruction of venous drainage or ischaemia due to hypotension may also contribute.

Prevention

Prevention should be along similar lines as for myopathy. This should aim to allow adequate perfusion and careful positioning to prevent abnormal pressures or tensions on nerve fibres. The hindlimbs should not be pulled out behind the horse with any force as this may predispose to femoral nerve paralysis. Headcollars should be removed when the horse is in lateral recumbency so that pressure on the facial nerve is avoided. Positioning to prevent triceps myopathy is appropriate to reduce pressure on the lower radial nerve. When prolonged surgery on any area is anticipated it is important to pay particular attention to the padding and support of the underlying tissues, as they may receive additional and prolonged pressure.

Treatment

Treatment is largely symptomatic, as the damage has already been done. In the recumbent case, management is similar to that for the horse with myopathy.

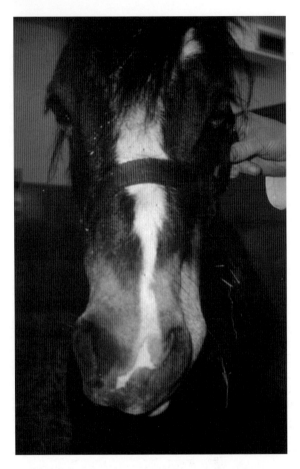

FIG 7.23 Facial paralysis after anaesthesia in lateral recumbency.

Support in slings may be particularly beneficial if the horse will tolerate them. Analgesics and sedatives may not be required and treatment is aimed more at reducing any suspected neural oedema. This includes NSAIDs at standard doses dexamethasone (2 mg/kg), and DMSO (1 g/kg by IV infusion).

SPINAL CORD MALACIA

The most serious postanaesthetic neuropathy is spinal cord malacia. This is not common but is always fatal. As with myopathy and other neuropathy, no sign is seen until the horse tries to stand up during recovery, or occasionally a few hours later.

Clinical signs

It is usually seen in large, young horses (particularly Shires) that have been anaesthetised in dorsal recumbency using volatile agents. The anaesthetic period may be relatively short and uneventful. Smaller horses, and very occasionally those positioned in lateral recumbency, have been affected. The horse usually develops flaccid paralysis from low thoracic or high lumbar segments so that the hindlimbs are affected. The horse make a few attempts to stand and often adopts a dog-sitting position, with the hindlimbs straightened out under the body (Figure 7.24). The animal is not usually

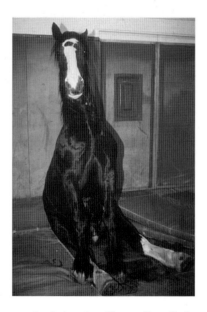

FIG 7.24 Spinal cord malacia. The horse commonly adopts a dog-sitting position with the hindlimbs positioned pointing straight forward. This horse is paralysed from the midlumbar region and is unable to rise. (Photograph courtesy of Dr GM Johnston.)

distressed, presumably because there is little pain associated with the condition. Some of these horses remain mentally alert and appear contented, eating and drinking readily (Figure 7.25). However, they deteriorate over the first 24–48 hours. The prognosis is hopeless and the diagnosis usually clear several hours after anaesthesia. There are no records of any that have recovered, although precise diagnosis is not possible *ante mortem*.

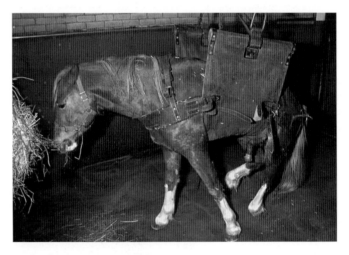

FIG 7.25 Spinal cord malacia. Horses with this condition rarely show signs of pain and may remain bright and alert for several days. This pony was comfortable and relaxed in slings, but never regained the use of its hindlimbs.

Pathogenesis

The pathogenesis remains a mystery, but is possibly associated with poor spinal cord perfusion, restricted venous drainage in the animal positioned in dorsal recumbency, or a vascular accident such a blood clot. Volatile anaesthetic hypotension can be expected to contribute to the ischaemia, although some cases have developed after anaesthesia where no hypotension occurred. It is possible that verminous arteritis may contribute to a poor arterial supply. It has also been suggested that Shire horses may have abnormal or deficient blood supply to the thoracolumbar spine, but there is no evidence to support this.

Prevention

It is difficult to recommend any preventative measures when the cause is unknown. However, since it appears that cord ischaemia from some source is the most likely cause, measures employed to prevent myopathy should also be appropriate for this condition. It is probably worth tilting any horse slightly off the vertical when it is anaesthetised in dorsal recumbency. This should prevent symmetrical occlusion of the spinal vascular supply or drainage and might ensure that some blood supply is maintained. This certainly seems worthwhile with a heavy horse, which is at the greatest risk.

EYE INJURY

During anaesthesia the normal protective blinking reflex is abolished and the cornea is vulnerable to damage. Ideally, anaesthesia should not be so deep that lacrimation ceases, but it is a wise precaution to place a film of non-medicated eye lubrication over the cornea once the horse is anaesthetised. This is especially important for the lower eye in a horse in lateral recumbency, or when the eyes are to be covered by surgical drapes. Care in positioning the head so that the eye is not compressed is essential (Figure 7.26). When head

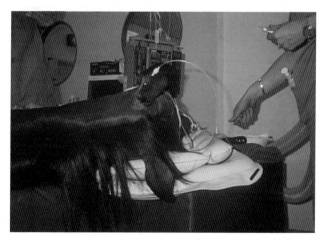

FIG 7.26 In lateral recumbency the head should be positioned so that the eye is not compressed against the table and does not lie in a pool of surgical scrub. The 'waffle' cushion illustrated here allows support of the head with the eye clear of any pressure.

surgery is to be performed, care is necessary to prevent cleansing agents used to prepare the surgical site from running into either eye. The lower eye should also be kept clear of any pool of cleansing agent that may collect during surgical preparation.

RECOVERY

Apart from the acute effects of anaesthetic agents on the cardiovascular and respiratory systems, most problems that occur in equine anaesthesia develop or become evident in the recovery period. Postoperative myopathy and neuropathy discussed above are the most obvious examples.

SELF-INFLICTED INJURY

Injury during recovery is a serious problem after anaesthesia in horses. It relates to their size, temperament, and the type and duration of surgery performed. The horse, presumably because it is essentially a flight animal that runs from anything that frightens or hurts it, commonly tries to stand before it is ready to do so. Major injury in the recovery period, particularly limb fractures necessitating euthanasia, causes a substantial number of the anaesthetic-related deaths in horses. A combination of ataxia and excitement is usually to blame. It is also probable that some horses which sustain a limb fracture in recovery may have been suffering from myopathy or neuropathy. Superficial injuries are not uncommon, particularly to periorbital tissues and the lips (Figure 7.27). These are usually mild and require only symptomatic treatment.

Prevention
It is impossible to guarantee an excitement- and ataxia-free recovery in every case. However, there are a number of measures that undoubtedly help to smooth this period.

Anaesthetic agents used. Induction and maintenance agents have some effect on the horse's behaviour in recovery. In general, slow recoveries tend to be calmer, and for this reason halothane may result in a better recovery than isoflurane. Sevoflurane is probably better than isoflurane, as although recovery is rapid, the horse tends to be calmer. Desflurane, with its very rapid recovery, has the advantage that the transition from unconsciousness to full control is very short. Sedation (see below) is recommended for recovery from

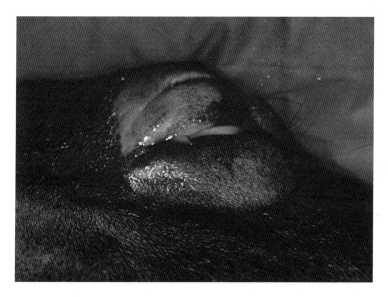

FIG 7.27 Superficial injuries to periorbital tissue occurred during a violent recovery.

these less soluble agents, or the horse may be disorientated by the rapidity of the return to consciousness. There is no doubt that recovery is better when only small doses of barbiturates have been used (up to 5 mg/kg thiopental) and some evidence that α_2 agonist–ketamine or α_2 agonist–thiopental induction lead to better recovery than guaiphenesin–thiopental. After long operations (more than 2 hours) the induction agent probably has little effect.

Analgesia. Good postoperative analgesia improves the behaviour of the horse in recovery. A horse that is in pain is far more likely to thrash around and attempt to get up too soon. One of the best forms of analgesia in the recovery period is good support of the injured site. Movement causes pain, and if the injury is well immobilised the degree of pain experienced when the horse starts to move may be reduced. If analgesics are given after surgery this should be before the horse regains consciousness or any beneficial effect on recovery will be lost. If analgesics are given after surgery, opioids given IM around 20 minutes before the end of anaesthesia are effective and can be given with NSAIDs if pain is likely to be severe (see Chapter 6). Regional nerve blocks can be used where proprioception will not be adversely affected. Perineural or intra-articular bupivacaine as appropriate, placed before surgery, improves the quality of surgical anaesthesia and provides postoperative analgesia (Chapter 6).

Quiet environment. Any disturbance during recovery is likely to upset a horse and encourage it to stand too soon. The animal must be watched during recovery, but it is important that it is not disturbed until obviously capable of standing. Low lighting helps to reduce stimulation at this stage.

Good surface. It appears that if the horse finds it difficult to get into sternal recumbency it may accept the restraint and lie still until it can make the necessary effort. For this reason, many clinics use deep, squashy mats for recovery. The horse certainly appears comfortable, but some system for their removal when the horse needs to walk is necessary. If mats are not used it is essential that the horse is allowed to recover on a surface that provides a degree of comfort, and a good grip is essential in all circumstances. A number of non-slip rubberised surfaces are available for purpose-built recovery boxes and are worth the expense. A good grass surface is ideal if weather and accessibility permit.

Position of horse in recovery box. Opinion differs as to whether the recovering horse should be turned on to the side that was uppermost during surgery. Undoubtedly, the horse is better able to stand if the operated leg is uppermost, and this should be the deciding factor. If the horse is turned, it must be very slowly; products of anaerobic metabolism will be released into the circulation and the lower lung and great vessels in the thorax will be compressed by the originally lower and now-oedematous lung. Hypoxaemia may be exacerbated, but previously compressed muscle will be perfused again more quickly. If there is no surgical reason otherwise, horses that have been in dorsal recumbency are best recovered right side up, as the right lung is larger.

Horses are less likely to injure themselves if they recover in a small padded box, as there is less space to develop any momentum. As long as a clear airway is assured, recovery may actually be improved if the horse rolls into an awkward position, as it will then be unable to stand until it has regained more consciousness and is stronger (Figure 7.28). Placing the horse with the head in a corner of the recovery box makes use of this fact.

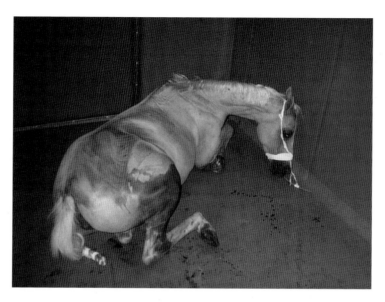

FIG 7.28 Although this horse appears to be in an awkward position in the recovery box it may actually benefit. As long as the airway is not obstructed and no extremities are awkwardly positioned, a horse placed in a corner is effectively better restrained and has to be strong and coordinated before it can stand. This may ultimately lead to better recovery.

Empty bladder. A horse with a full bladder is very restless and few will empty it before standing. Hence a full bladder leads to early and uncoordinated attempts to stand. After a long operation, particularly where α_2 agonists or large volumes of fluid have been given, it is extremely worthwhile emptying the bladder by catheterisation before recovery (Figure 7.29); better still, a catheter can be left in place throughout surgery to prevent any accumulation of urine.

Respiratory support. Nasal obstruction is not uncommon during recovery, particularly after a horse has been anaesthetised in dorsal recumbency, as the nasal mucosa becomes congested. This can be reduced if the head is raised and the neck slightly flexed at the pole to bring up the nose (Figure 7.30). This is similar to the position recommended to prevent laryngeal paralysis. When the

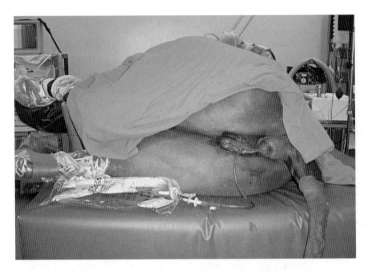

FIG 7.29 *The bladder should be catheterised for any prolonged surgery, especially if large doses of α_2 agonists are given.*

endotracheal tube is removed it is essential to ensure there is no obstruction to air movement. A nasal tube should be placed if there is any difficulty in breathing. A small cuffless endotracheal tube can be used; this should be taped in place and removed after the horse stands up (Figure 7.31a). Alternatively, a shorter nasal tube with a thick plastic end that prevents aspiration can be left in place without tape, and will fall out safely when the horse sits up or stands (Figure 7.31b). A further approach is to leave the endotracheal tube in place with the proximal end pulled out through the bar of the mouth, again secured with tape (Figure 7.32). Horses tolerate this very well and rarely cough, even as the tube is removed.

Hypoxaemia is likely to develop during recovery, as the horse is no longer inspiring a high oxygen fraction. Oxygen can be delivered via the nasal or endotracheal tube while the horse remains in lateral recumbency. Flow rates of at least 15 L/min are required to have any impact on the hypoxaemia, and are quite difficult to maintain when the horse starts to move. A demand valve (Figure 3.7, page 46) can be used to supply a higher oxygen fraction while the

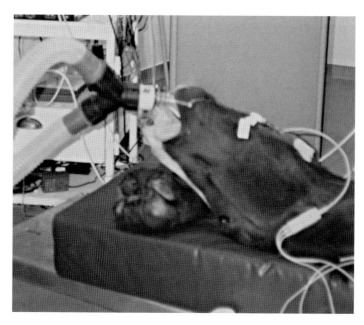

FIG 7.30 *The head is positioned with the neck slightly flexed to improve nasal venous drainage and prevent laryngeal nerve damage.*

endotracheal tube is in place but will depress respiration if used with spontaneous respiration, as it increases the work of breathing. Operated manually, the demand valve is the best way to supplement oxygen in a seriously hypoxic horse during recovery. Severe hypoxia causes marked restlessness, and horses that appear cyanotic and distressed should be given oxygen even if it is not routinely used in recovery.

Sedation. Sedation can be used to prolong the period that the horse remains lying down to try to calm the period between unconsciousness and readiness to stand. Xylazine in IV boluses of 50–100 mg is the most widely used. A more marked effect will be achieved if it is used in combination with opioid analgesics. Detomidine (0.001–0.002 mg/kg) has also been used, but may prolong the recovery more than the shorter-acting xylazine. Very small volumes

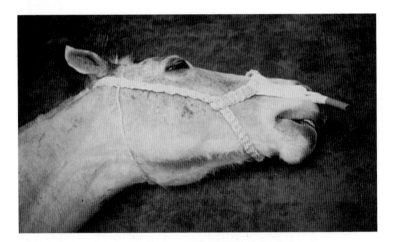

FIG 7.31a   A nasal tube should be placed and secured if there is any indication of respiratory obstruction when the endotracheal tube is removed. A small endotracheal tube can be securely taped in place.

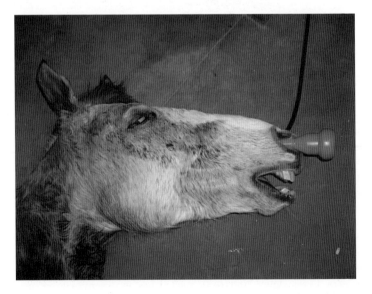

FIG 7.31b   Purpose-made nasal tubes with a bulbous end prevent the danger of inhalation.

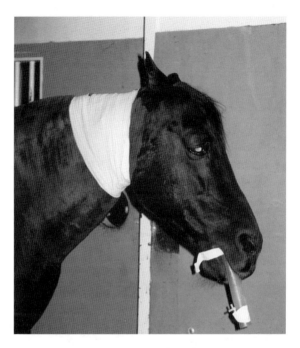

FIG 7.32 Horses tolerate an oral tracheal tube remarkably well, and in many clinics they are routinely recovered with an endotracheal tube in place. This horse has been standing for several minutes after recovery and did not cough at all.

are required, which makes dosing difficult. Romifidine (0.01–0.02 mg/kg) is also likely to prolong recovery. If not used in premedication, acepromazine may be useful at this stage as a mild calming agent. Immediately after anaesthesia only small doses of the α_2 agonists should be given; larger doses may be used later.

Manual support. Head and tail ropes, slings and swimming pools have all been used to assist the horse in recovery. Some control is essential after major orthopaedic surgery, where the surgical repair can be fatally ruined by one false move. Any system using rope support on the tail must be securely fastened (Figure 7.33a,b).

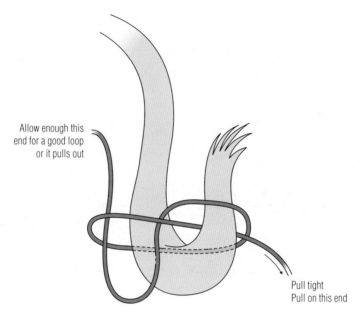

Allow enough this
end for a good loop
or it pulls out

Pull tight
Pull on this end

FIG 7.33a   Recommended method of tying the tail hitch.

A system using head and tail ropes pulled through rings high on the wall is probably the most practical, in that it allows assistance to be given in lifting the horse without risk of injury to handlers. This, particularly the tail rope, also helps to stabilize the horse after it has stood up. Such stabilisation helps to prevent accidents that occur after the horse has regained its feet before it has gained full control over its limbs. A technique developed by H. Wilderjans using climbing equipment has proved successful and can be performed by only one handler. Two handlers, one on the head and one on the tail, are best used for high-risk cases, such as horses recovering after repair of a long bone fracture. The rings used for this purpose must be bolted through the wall higher than a standing horse's head (around 2 m above the floor) (Figure 7.34a). Locking carabiners are placed on each ring so that the ropes run smoothly. An additional pulley on the tail rope ring further aids smooth traction. Two lengths each of at least 10 m of 8–9 mm diameter nylon mountaineering or sailing rope are attached, one each to head and tail and through the carabiner or pulley on the recovery box wall. Softer 10–12 mm rope, which is more

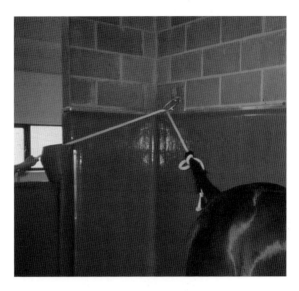

FIG 7.33b *When the tail hitch is pulled tight it is secure, as it tightens on itself.*

comfortable to hold, can be used on the head, but the tail rope must be 8–9 mm in diameter so that it runs easily through the grigri (see below). Different-coloured ropes for head and tail help to distinguish them when they are in use. An unbreakable nylon headcollar without bulky metal rings or buckles is essential; the head rope is attached to a ring at the front of the noseband (Figure 7.34b). The tail rope must be securely fastened (Figure 7.34c), as failure of either rope will lead to disaster. An emergency quick-release locking device (e.g. a Petzl grigri) is used on the tail rope outside the recovery box (Figure 7.34d) so that one person can control the tail rope of any size of horse. The tail rope can thus be locked to assist in holding the tail, but may also be released quickly if necessary. Depending on the size of the recovery room, the handler stands either inside or outside the recovery box. The ropes are generally pulled through a small opening in the box door (Figure 7.34e). The tail rope must be on maximum tension when the horse is still lying down. When the horse starts to stand, the assistant helps to lift its hindquarters by pulling on the tail rope. The head is controlled but not pulled up. Once the horse is standing, both head and tail ropes should stabilise and support it against a wall of the recovery room until it can stand unaided without ataxia

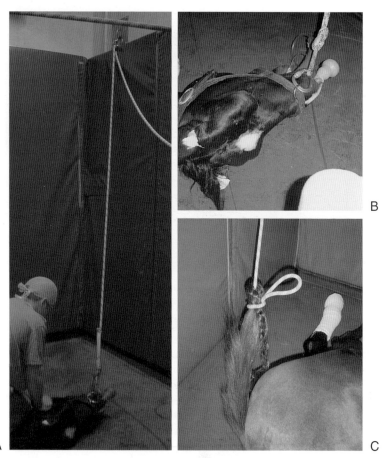

FIG 7.34a, b & c (A) The wall rings used for assisted recovery must be securely bolted through the wall around 2 m above the floor. (B) An unbreakable nylon headcollar is used for assisted recovery. The head rope is attached to a ring at the front of the noseband. (C) The tail rope must be securely fastened, as failure will lead to disaster

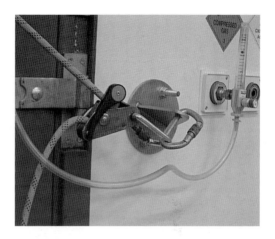

FIG 7.34d A Petzl grigri emergency quick-release locking device is used on the tail rope outside the recovery box.

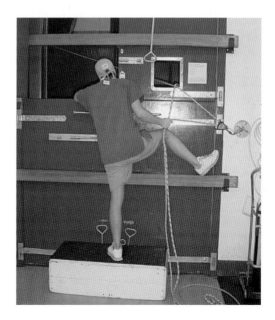

FIG 7.34e The rops can be pulled by one person through a small opening in the recovery box door.

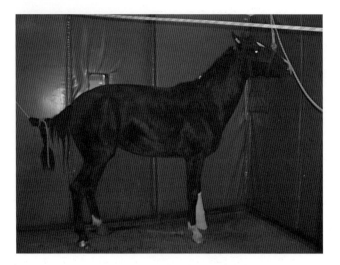

FIG 7.34f   *Head and tail ropes are used to stabilise and support the horse until it has regained muscle strength and can stand unaided without danger of falling over.*

and has regained muscle strength (Figure 7.34f). The horse should not be left unattended while attached to the ropes.

The technique needs to be learned and practised for smooth and reliable operation. It should not be reserved only for high-risk cases, so that when assisted recovery is essential the handlers are familiar with the process and understand how best to use it. It is undoubtedly best learned from a clinic that routinely uses the system.

It is undoubtedly of considerable benefit to keep the horse in lateral recumbency until judged ready to stand, so that it does not attempt to stand until it is able to do so at the first attempt. Judicious sedation is required as described above; one handler can then kneel behind the horse's head with a knee on the neck and raise the horse's nose when it attempts to struggle (Figure 7.35). It is rarely necessary to keep the horse lying down for longer than an hour before letting it attempt to stand. Actual duration is anaesthetic agent-dependent; some attempt should be made to judge whether it is ready.

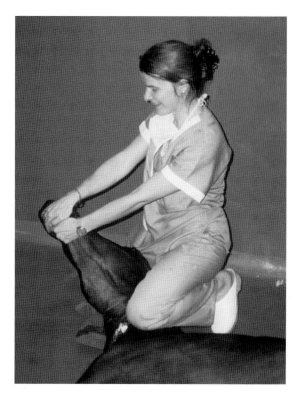

FIG 7.35 *A horse can be restrained in lateral recumbency if the nose is raised while pressure is applied to the neck with a knee. This prevents the horse from swinging its head ventrally, which is essential for it to move into sternal recumbency and try to stand.*

Return of normal tongue tone is often a good indication that the limb muscles are ready for the attempt. At this point the head and tail assistance described above is brought into play.

If head and tail ropes are not available, the horse may be left to stand on its own; alternatively, some attempt can be made to assist its efforts. This carries a high risk of injury to handlers and should not be attempted without experienced personnel, adequate space, and an escape route for people. It is

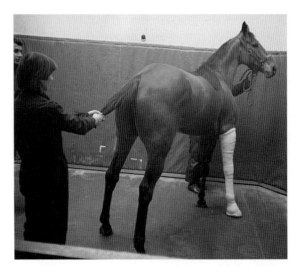

FIG 7.36 This horse was allowed to stand by himself, but once on his feet was restrained at head and tail to prevent him from walking until he had regained good control of his limbs.

extremely difficult to support any animal larger than a pony in this way, although support at the head and on the tail as the animal stands up is of some benefit without ropes. There is no doubt that there is great benefit in supporting the horse immediately after it stands (Figure 7.36). The horse should be made to stand still, and preferably be supported against a wall while it reorientates and gains muscle strength. There should be one person at the head and one holding the tail at this stage. The horse should then be allowed to stand until it is willing and able to walk forward without danger of falling over. Occasionally a horse may become very excited and difficult to manage immediately after standing; further α_2 agonist sedation, with butorphanol if necessary, is essential at this stage to prevent injury to both personnel and the horse itself.

POSTOPERATIVE COLIC

General anaesthesia depresses gut motility and development of postoperative colic is not unusual. This ranges from transient mild discomfort and reduced passage of faeces to caecal impaction, which may lead to fatal rupture.

Starvation depresses gut motility and may predispose to this condition. The α_2 agonists also have a marked depressant effect on gut motility, although they do not appear to be associated with a greater incidence of postoperative colic. Intravenous penicillin (sodium and potassium salts) appears to induce the passage of liquid faeces and may contribute to an overall imbalance of the control of gut motility. Perioperative opioids, particularly morphine, may predispose towards postoperative colic. The precise aetiology of postoperative colic is not understood, though it is likely to be multifactorial; it remains another, if minor, hazard of equine anaesthesia. The horse should be prevented from eating large quantities of roughage in the immediate postoperative period so that any intestinal hypomotility does not lead to impaction.

CARDIAC ARREST AND RESUSCITATION (TABLE 7.1)

The term 'cardiac arrest' is used to describe the situation when the heart no longer has any output. Cardiac arrest occurs in anaesthetised horses for a variety of reasons, sometimes due to the pathological condition of the horse, but sometimes in otherwise apparently healthy animals. Possible reasons for the latter include changes in autonomic control (most commonly through vagal stimulation, leading to asystole) and anaesthetic-induced myocardial depression and hypotension. Some cases appear to be idiopathic, and cardiac arrest can occur with no prior warning. The three main forms of arrest are asystole, ventricular fibrillation, and electromechanical dissociation. In horses not suffering from any metabolic disease the heart usually stops in asystole, any period of fibrillation being transient. In toxic horses ventricular tachycardia may precede a definite period of ventricular fibrillation, but asystole usually follows rapidly; use of defibrillators is rarely, if ever, necessary.

Contrary to what is often stated, in the authors' experience horses not suffering from any serious metabolic disorders but that suffer cardiac arrest during anaesthesia can be resuscitated effectively in about 50% of cases, utilising the simple routine outlined below (Table 7.1). In such cases, if the heart can be restarted and regain spontaneous rhythm there appear to be few after-effects and overall survival is good, the horse returning to normal activities. However, success depends on speed of detection. If the horse is 'brain dead' before the arrest is noted, there is no chance of its survival.

Table 7.1 Routine for cardiopulmonary resuscitation (CPR) after cardiac arrest

Stage 1 – Immediate action

Tell surgeon/try to get extra help. Assign responsibilities

Look at the clock and note the time.

External cardiac massage: 20–30 per minute

Horse in lateral recumbency with the front leg drawn forward – on a hard surface if possible.

Cardiac massage is performed by jumping on the horse's chest in the kneeling position.

Stop giving more anaesthetic.

Clear and maintain airway. IPPV with oxygen

Endotracheal intubation.

IPPV even if the horse is apparently still breathing itself.

This routine provides adequate blood flow and oxygenation of vital tissues while drugs are found and drawn up.

The success of cardiac massage is judged by the continuation of signs that there is still oxygenation of the brain, i.e. nystagmus, corneal reflex, sometimes agonal gasping, even normal respiration. If the arterial blood pressure line is still in place, then efficacy can be assessed. There will be an end-tidal CO_2 but it will be low.

Stage 2 – Drug treatment

Drugs must not be given until cardiac massage provides adequate blood flow.

Asystole (commonest in anaesthetised horses)

Adrenaline IV. Continue massage and IPPV.

Adrenaline dose **0.3 mL/100 kg** of 1:1000 (= 0.003 mg/kg).

If that fails,

Atropine or glycopyrrolate IV. Continue massage and IPPV.

Atropine dose: **1.6 mL/100 kg of 0.6 mg/mL** = 0.01 mg/kg.

Glycopyrrolate dose: **2.5 mL/100 kg of 0.2 mg/mL** = 0.005 mg/kg.

If that fails,

Adrenaline IV. Continue massage and IPPV.

Adrenaline dose **0.5 mL/100 kg** of 1:000 (= 0.005 mg/kg).

Ventricular fibrillation

Very unusual in the horse.

Defibrillate if equipment available.

Lidocaine IV. Continue massage and IPPV.

Lidocaine dose: **2.5 mL/100 kg of 20 mg/mL** (= 0.5 mg/kg)

Stage 3

Once spontaneous rhythm is restored, treatment depends on the state of the horse as well as the original cause of the problem. Heart rhythm and hypotension may need treatment (pages 79–81). If anticholinergics have been used, very small doses of dobutamine should be given or severe tachycardia will occur (page 80). Causes of the original arrest, where known, should be corrected as far as possible.

Table 7.1 Routine for cardiopulmonary resuscitation (CPR) after cardiac arrest—cont'd

Notes on the recommended routine

Cardiac massage

Cardiac massage in the horse can be very effective, but it is exhausting and no one person can keep it up effectively for much more than 5 minutes. The effort needed depends on the size of the horse and the weight of the person carrying out resuscitation. A small person resuscitating a large horse may have to use all their strength, but a large person reviving a small pony does not have to use full force. It is not necessary to break the horse's ribs (although this may happen, and is preferable to a dead horse). In the absence of a working arterial pressure line, efficacy of cardiac massage is judged by the maintenance of central nervous reflexes.

Duration of resuscitation

If the horse was in good health prior to anaesthesia, the basic resuscitative measures outlined above should be continued for as long as it still shows signs of brain activity. The authors have successfully resuscitated a pony following 25 minutes of such treatment!

Drug doses

Drugs required for resuscitation (adrenaline (epinephrine), lidocaine, anticholinergics) should be available in an 'emergency box' and, for easy dosage, should be labelled in 'mL per weight' of the actual solutions kept in the box.

Post-resuscitation treatment

Post-resuscitation treatment aims to correct acidosis and to prevent pulmonary and cerebral oedema, which may occur as a result of tissue oxygen deprivation. Agents used include bicarbonate, diuretics and corticosteroids. If detection of cardiac arrest and the application of effective basic CPR has been rapid, then there should be minimal tissue damage; serious post-resuscitation problems in the horse are rare

DETECTION OF CARDIAC ARREST IN THE HORSE

Without electronic monitoring this is virtually impossible to do quickly enough. It is impossible to palpate a pulse, mucous membranes are grey and capillary refill time very slow, all features that may be seen under volatile agent anaesthesia without cardiac arrest. During cardiac arrest no heartbeat can be auscultated, but surgery often prevents easy access to the chest.

One of the greatest problems is that, following cardiac arrest, the horse 'appears to be waking up'. The eye may show nystagmus, the horse blinks and it will usually continue breathing. Sometimes the breathing becomes agonal, with the effect that the limbs jerk, giving the impression that the horse is waking up and moving; the common response is thus to increase the anaesthetic vaporiser setting. By the time the signs disappear the horse is 'brain dead' and resuscitation is unlikely to be successful.

With adequate electronic monitoring (Chapter 5) cardiac arrest can be easily detected by the ECG trace, unless it is in electromechanical dissociation. The arterial blood pressure trace will be low and flat (it does not always fall to zero) and end-tidal carbon dioxide will fall sharply. However, monitors may fail, and the condition of the horse, particularly the presence or absence of a palpable pulse, should be checked before active resuscitation is started.

RESUSCITATION

The routine for cardiopulmonary resuscitation (CPR) as applied to anaesthetised horses in an equine theatre is shown in Table 7.1. (stages 1 & 2 are appropriate for posting as the theatre wall)

Further reading

Borer KE and Clarke KW (2006) The effect of hyoscine on dobutamine requirement in spontaneously breathing horses anaesthetized with halothane. *Veterinary Anaesthesia and Analgesia* **33**: 149–157

Castillo S and Matthews NS (2005) How to assemble, apply and use a head and tail rope system for the recovery of the equine anaesthetic patient. Proceedings of the 51st Annual Convention of the AAEP, 490.

Grandy JL, Steffey EP, Hodgson DS, et al (1987) Arterial hypotension and the development of postanesthetic myopathy in halothane-anesthetized horses. *American Journal of Veterinary Research* **48**: 92–197.

Hall LW, Clarke KW and Trim CM (2001) *Veterinary Anaesthesia*, 10th edn. WB Saunders, London.

Johnston GM, Eastment JK, Taylor PM and Wood JLN (2002) The confidential enquiry of perioperative equine fatalities (CEPEF-1): mortality results of phases 1 and 2. *Veterinary Anaesthesia and Analgesia* **29**: 159–170.

Johnston GM, Eastment JK, Taylor PM, et al (2004) Is isoflurane safer than halothane in equine anaesthesia? Results from a prospective multicentre randomised controlled trial. *Equine Veterinary Journal* **36**: 64–71.

Lindsay WA, Robinson GM, Brunson DB, et al (1989) Induction of equine postanesthetic myositis after halothane-induced hypotension. *American Journal of Veterinary Research* **50**: 404–410.

Lindsay WA, McDonell WN and Bignell W (1980) Equine postanesthetic forelimb lameness: intracompartmental pressure changes and biochemical patterns. *American Journal of Veterinary Research* **41**: 1919–1192.

McGurrin MKJ and Physick-Sheard PW (2005) A review of treatment options and prognosis in equine atrial fibrillation. Proceedings of the 51st Annual Convention of the AAEP, 149–152.

Muir WW and Hubbell JAE (1991) *Muir and Hubbell's Equine Anaesthesia: Monitoring and Emergency Therapy.* Mosby Year Book, St Louis, 419–443, 461–484.

Raisis AL (2005) Skeletal muscle blood flow in anaesthetized horses. Part I: effects of anaesthetics and vasoactive agents. *Veterinary Anaesthesia and Analgesia* **32**: 324–330

Raisis AL (2005) Skeletal muscle blood flow in anaesthetized horses. Part II: effects of anaesthetics and vasoactive agents. *Veterinary Anaesthesia and Analgesia* **32**: 331–337.

Taylor PM and Young SS (1990) The effect of limb position on venous and compartmental pressure in the forelimb of ponies. *Journal of the Association of Veterinary Anaesthetists* **17**: 35–37.

Wagner AE, Bednarski RM and Muir WW (1990) Hemodynamic effects of carbon dioxide during intermittent positive pressure ventilation in horses. *American Journal of Veterinary Research* **51**: 1922–1928.

Young SS and Taylor PM (1993) Factors influencing the outcome of equine anaesthesia: a review of 1,314 cases. *Equine Veterinary Journal* **25**: 147–151.

8

ANAESTHESIA IN SPECIAL SITUATIONS

The main aim of anaesthesia for a special case is to 'give the best anaesthetic you can'. This of course applies to any procedure; however, the high-risk case has less tolerance for mistakes as it has less reserve. A 'low-risk' case (no horse is truly low risk) can withstand a few man-made mistakes, although it is better that they do not happen. There are a number of features about some conditions that require special attention, and these are outlined below. Common conditions or those of particular interest in equine anaesthesia are described.

Equine anaesthesia contrasts with that in humans and small domestic species in that, with one notable exception (the horse with colic), virtually all patients presenting for anaesthesia are healthy. The greatest challenge to the equine anaesthetist is the healthy athlete who presents for elective orthopaedic surgery or for repair of an acute injury. Part of the difficulty is the psychological (and practical) requirement that the healthy horse should remain healthy. Anything that happens to it subsequently is the fault of the treatment (or anaesthesia). The very best the anaesthetist can do is return it to the state in which it started; anything else is worse.

FIT, ATHLETIC HORSE

All competition horses are athletes, even if they have been 'let down' before elective surgery. The top-class flat-racing Thoroughbred is the most difficult of them all.

PATHOPHYSIOLOGY
The athlete has enormous cardiovascular and respiratory reserve. At rest and during anaesthesia energy requirements are low and only baseline function is required; heart and respiratory rates may be very low. Anaesthesia, which reduces cardiac and respiratory stimulation and causes overt depression, makes matters worse. Apnoea or marked bradypnoea (below 7 per minute) is common in the healthy anaesthetised Thoroughbred even in the face of hypercapnia. Bradycardia (below 25 per minute) is also common and does not respond to surgical stimulation. Coupled with anaesthetic agent-induced

myocardial depression the result is low cardiac output, hypotension and severe respiratory acidosis. The athlete's heart is large and itself needs adequate blood pressure to ensure that perfusion of the myocardium is sufficient. Hence severe anaesthetic-induced cardiovascular depression may have disastrous consequences.

GENERAL PRINCIPLES OF MANAGEMENT

The horse is healthy and there is no disease to treat. Handling should be calm but firm to settle a restless horse, and low doses of acepromazine are appropriate both to relax the horse and to decrease the risk of cardiovascular catastrophe. The surgical area should be clipped beforehand to reduce the duration of anaesthesia. In elective cases this can be done on the previous day, under sedation if necessary.

Athletic horses are sensitive to volatile anaesthetics and may develop severe hypotension even when anaesthesia is not deep enough for surgery. It is difficult to believe that a horse kicking in response to surgery may be hypotensive unless the blood pressure is measured. It is essential that arterial blood pressure monitoring starts as soon as possible after induction of anaesthesia. Means of supporting the circulation with fluids and inotropes should be made ready before induction. If hypotension develops when anaesthesia is inadequate, cardiac support with intravenous fluids and inotropes should start immediately (pages 79–81) and supplementary intravenous agents given (pages 77–79) instead of increasing the inspired anaesthetic concentration.

Apnoea is common in horses immediately after induction whatever the agent used, and if prolonged surgery (more than 60–90 minutes) is anticipated it may be judicious to start intermittent positive-pressure ventilation (IPPV) immediately after induction. This smoothes the transition to the volatile agent as it is taken up more consistently than with the horse's irregular attempts at respiration. Unfortunately, IPPV enhances cardiovascular depression because more anaesthetic agent is taken up and raised intrathoracic pressures reduce venous return.

Isoflurane is usually considered a better agent than halothane to use in the athletic horse (see Chapter 4). It has been shown that the risk of death from cardiovascular causes is less with isoflurane than with halothane in the young healthy adult (2–5-year-old). Sevoflurane and desflurane have not been examined in this way.

ELECTIVE ORTHOPAEDIC SURGERY

Orthopaedic surgery is often performed in fit, athletic horses and the points raised above obviously also apply.

PREOPERATIVE PREPARATION

Few horses presenting for elective orthopaedic surgery are in a great deal of pain. However, it is likely that surgery will cause postoperative pain, and administration of an analgesic as part of the premedication should improve postoperative analgesia through a pre-emptive effect (see Chapter 6). A NSAID is often appropriate before arthroscopic surgery and is given at the same time as premedication. Where more invasive surgery is anticipated an opioid may be included (Chapter 6), and this will also enhance the effect of sedative premedication. Background 'analgesia' during surgery may smooth the course of anaesthesia.

ANAESTHESIA

Induction of anaesthesia is potentially hazardous for any horse with a limb injury, although this is more significant with acute trauma (page 180). If the limb is unstable it should be supported in a cast or Robert Jones bandage and induction should be assisted (pages 124–129). As surgery may be prolonged, extreme care with positioning is important.

The considerations for the athletic horse outlined above apply to most animals undergoing orthopaedic surgery. In the face of a substantial surgical stimulus it may be difficult to maintain an adequate depth of anaesthesia without excessive cardiorespiratory depression. Supplementary intravenous agents are often required. Local anaesthesia is particularly relevant for orthopaedic cases as described previously (Chapter 6). During arthroscopic surgery surgical stimulation may be very limited and it is sometimes difficult to maintain adequate cardiovascular function because of the lack of stimulation. Sudden movement in such cases may be a disaster and must be avoided. Neuromuscular blockade may be particularly valuable under both these conditions (pages 81–84). Some procedures may be prolonged, and careful monitoring of cardiovascular and respiratory systems is vital. It is often easiest to run such anaesthetics by maximum interference with IPPV and cardiac support from the start. Even if cardiorespiratory system function is good at the beginning of anaesthesia, it may deteriorate; it is easier to maintain the status quo than to retrieve cardiac and respiratory function when it is severely depressed. Although the cardiovascular merits of isoflurane may make it an appropriate choice over halothane for these cases, the more abrupt recovery from isoflurane is often considered a disadvantage when a vulnerable surgical repair is at stake. The choice of agents in this case is down to personal choice and experience, and sevoflurane is now often chosen to replace halothane. In the future desflurane may prove another alternative.

RECOVERY

Recovery from anaesthesia is often the most critical part of orthopaedic surgery. If major surgery has been performed, resulting in a potentially fragile limb whose surgical repair can easily be destroyed, it is essential to use some form of assisted recovery (pages 163–170). After most arthroscopic surgery it is not necessary to assist recovery as it unlikely that the repair will be damaged. A smooth, controlled recovery is, of course, still the aim.

The most difficult recoveries to manage are those with a horse in a full-length hindlimb cast (Figure 8.1). The horse generally dislikes and is frightened by any dressing over the hock, and most do not know how to handle the full-length cast. Each must be managed according to its own temperament, but it is most important that the animal is not allowed to attempt to stand before it is judged to be ready. The authors believe, from their experience, that these cases should always be assisted to some degree (pages 163–170). A full forelimb cast causes some of the same problems, but most horses manage them better.

ACUTE TRAUMA

In horses, anaesthesia for repair of acute traumatic injury usually involves orthopaedic surgery and is often in the fit athlete. Hence, most of the considerations for athletic horses and orthopaedic surgery outlined above also apply.

PATHOPHYSIOLOGY

The acute case is often restless and distressed, sometimes to the point of overt excitement. Pain from the injury undoubtedly contributes to this. Circulating catecholamines are high and the horse tends to be difficult to handle.

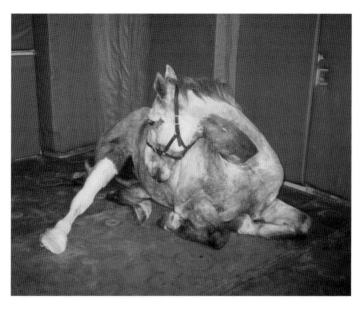

FIG 8.1 A horse with a full length hindlimb cast is the most difficult to recover from anaesthesia. The horse does not tolerate the restriction well. Slight flexion in the cast is beneficial, and the animal should be placed with the affected leg uppermost so that it may push off from the good leg when trying to stand. Assistance with head and tail ropes is extremely worthwhile in such cases.

There may have been substantial blood loss, and it is likely that the horse will be dehydrated owing both to strenuous exercise and a long period since it last ate or drank. All these contribute to an unstable cardiovascular system.

Dehydration. The dehydration present in the acute case that has been admitted immediately after strenuous work rarely needs preoperative treatment, but generous quantities of intravenous crystalloids should be given during surgery. The truly exhausted horse with heat stroke certainly needs stabilising before anaesthesia. These cases should not be given phenothiazines until near normovolaemia has been restored or very severe hypotension may ensue.

Blood loss. Theoretically, a horse that has lost a substantial amount of blood, for instance in a road traffic accident, should have the circulating volume restored before anaesthesia. The exception to this rule is where anaesthesia is necessary to stem the source of bleeding. The volume of blood lost from apparently small wounds below the fetlock, and also from guttural pouch mycosis, may be deceptively large, and phenothiazines should not be given as the resulting hypotension may make the horse faint. Such loss is ideally replaced with a colloid so that it stays in the circulation. However, this is rarely feasible in the horse, although hydroxyethyl starches and the gelatine-based products have been used successfully. Isotonic crystalloid solutions such as Ringer's lactate are generally given. Three times the volume of blood lost is required, as crystalloids spread throughout the extracellular fluid (ECF) and do not remain in the circulation. It may be difficult to estimate the volume of blood lost, and the signs will depend on how rapidly it has been lost. However, it is unlikely that any obvious sign of hypovolaemia will be seen if the horse has lost less than 10% of its circulating blood volume. Thus 10% (approximately 5 L in a 500 kg horse, plus 10 L to allow for the shift to the ECF) can first be given as fast as possible; the effects are monitored, and more is given according to the response of pulse rate and quality, mucous membrane colour, demeanour and urinary output. Hypertonic saline (4 mL/kg of 7.5% solution) can be used if the circulation is collapsed. This must be followed up with isotonic electrolytes to restore the ECF, but is initially life saving in the face of severe depletion of circulating blood volume.

Analgesia. Good pain management is essential in the horse with acute traumatic injury (see Chapter 6). It is appropriate in most of these cases to combine opioids and NSAIDs. Good analgesia will calm the horse, greatly easing preoperative preparation such as radiography. However good the analgesia, pain will not be entirely removed and the risk that analgesia will cause the horse to weight-bear suddenly and cause more damage to an unstable limb is largely hypothetical. If the horse becomes ataxic there is a risk of further injury, and large doses of the α_2 agonists should not be given until the horse is standing where anaesthesia is to be induced. Good support of an injured limb in a cast or Robert Jones bandage is essential for induction, when further injury may occur as the horse becomes unconscious and loses control of its limbs. Good support of the injury also enhances analgesia and calms the horse by giving it confidence in its ability to walk. Low doses of acepromazine can be used in horses that are not dehydrated. This will enhance the calming effect of analgesia without causing ataxia.

ANAESTHESIA
Induction and recovery
As for the elective orthopaedic case, some means of assisting induction and recovery (pages 124–129, 163–170) is essential if the injury has destabilised a limb. Further damage at induction may make surgery impossible; equally, a violent recovery can easily destroy the repair.

Maintenance
Anaesthesia for acute orthopaedic injury is often more straightforward than for elective orthopaedic surgery, as the trauma and pain-induced sympathetic stimulation present before induction may prevent bradycardia and apnoea. However, all the potential hazards outlined above still apply and maximum support is required throughout. Fracture repair is often prolonged, good positioning is essential, and the cardiovascular and respiratory systems must be supported throughout. Neuromuscular blockade (pages 81–84) is particularly valuable in such cases, especially during reduction of the fracture and until it is stabilised. There is still plenty of time thereafter to ensure complete reversal.

Although horses undergoing surgery for acute trauma sustained during exercise or competition would appear to carry a greater anaesthetic risk, most formal investigations of the pathophysiology and clinical outcome of such cases suggest that horses tolerate this remarkably well. It has been suggested that they may be more likely to develop postoperative myopathy as a result of low-grade muscle injury from the exercise. High circulating catecholamines and a hypermetabolic state may also contribute. It is particularly important that these horses do not suffer further muscle injury, and careful attention to the preventative measures outlined on pages 142–146 is mandatory.

CHEST INJURY
Surgery for repair of acute trauma other than orthopaedic injury is uncommon in the horse. However, chest injury, usually from a stake wound or a road traffic accident, has a number of special considerations. Management of blood loss and pain is as described above. The main consideration in chest injury is the mechanical effect on respiration. If the chest has been penetrated, the hole must be covered to prevent lung collapse during preparation for anaesthesia. Once the horse is anaesthetised, IPPV must be employed while the injury is repaired. Even if the chest was not penetrated before surgery it is highly likely that this will happen during surgical repair, and means of

supplying IPPV must be readily available should this occur. If no ventilator is available and there are no extra willing pairs of hands to ventilate, manually, a horse with a chest injury should be referred to a centre that has the necessary equipment.

Other than the mechanical effect of opening the chest wall, anaesthesia for repair of chest injury does not present many other specific problems. It is conceivable that bradycardia may occur if the vagus nerve trunk is stimulated during exploration of the chest. This should be treated with anticholinergics, such as glycopyrrolate (0.005 mg/kg) or atropine (0.005–0.01 mg/kg). A chest drain must be placed before the incision is closed in order to remove air and fluid from the chest before spontaneous respiration returns. Some lung collapse is inevitable, and supplementary oxygen should be supplied at least until the horse is in sternal recumbency. It is pertinent to recover the horse with the endotracheal tube in place. Postoperative analgesia is essential: thoracic pain decreases chest wall excursion, leading to impaired respiratory function. Local intercostal nerve blocks provide excellent postoperative analgesia.

HEAD INJURY

Occasionally horses require anaesthesia and surgery to lift a depressed cranial fracture. In practice, horses presented for surgery rarely have signs of serious neurological dysfunction and most can be treated as any other horse with an acute injury.

The aim in anaesthesia of the head-injured patient is to prevent any further rise in intracerebral pressure and maintain sufficient blood flow to the whole brain. In theory, the drugs commonly used for anaesthesia in horses, such as α_2 agonists, ketamine and volatile agents, are not ideal. However, the value of a smooth, calm induction and recovery cannot be overstated; if otherwise unsuitable drugs lead to calm induction and recovery this is good justification for their use. Maintenance of adequate cerebral perfusion is important, so maintenance of good circulatory function is essential; the usual methods (pages 77–81) are employed. Hypercapnia should be avoided as this increases cerebral perfusion and raises intracranial pressure. IPPV should be employed in these cases; even a horse that appears to be breathing well is likely to be hypercapnic. Isoflurane and sevoflurane are certainly preferable to halothane, as their effects on cerebral circulation are more appropriate.

SURGERY FOR COLIC

PATHOPHYSIOLOGY

The horse with colic represents a wide range of physiological states. Surgery is generally required to relieve a physical or functional obstruction of the intestine. The obstruction upsets normal fluid and electrolyte homoeostasis, and the ECF is depleted as fluid moves into the proximal part of the gut but is not reabsorbed further on. Once the gut wall is damaged extra fluid is excreted into the gut lumen, so massive volumes can be lost from the ECF and the circulation. The fluid loss is essentially isotonic, so there is little osmotic shift between ICF and ECF. The ECF (which includes the circulation) is a relatively small compartment, so dehydration and cardiovascular collapse soon occur. The situation is made worse by the direct effect of endotoxaemia on capillary integrity, resulting in further massive fluid loss out of the circulation into the tissues. Additional insult occurs as distended bowel puts pressure through the diaphragm on to thoracic structures, causing respiratory embarrassment and exacerbating the cardiovascular collapse. The obstruction also causes pain due to distension of and damage to the bowel wall.

PREOPERATIVE MANAGEMENT

Premedication and analgesia

Analgesia is required on humanitarian grounds, for the safety of both horse and operators, and to allow preparation for surgery. α_2 agonists are excellent visceral analgesics as well as sedatives and are extremely useful in these circumstances. Xylazine (0.25–0.5 mg/kg) is the shortest acting, but low doses of detomidine (0.005–0.01 mg/kg) or romifidine (0.025–0.05 mg/kg) are also used. The α_2 agonists depress heart rate and gut motility and must therefore be used with care. High doses should be avoided.

NSAIDs, such as flunixin (1 mg/kg), should be given once the decision has been made to operate. NSAIDs protect against the effects of endotoxin and are indicated for surgery. Endotoxin may be released during surgery, for instance when strangulated bowel is unravelled, and some of the depressant effects on the cardiovascular system will be obtunded if flunixin is already present.

Short-acting opioids such as butorphanol or pethidine are also suitable analgesics. They have little effect on the cardiovascular system and are excellent premedicants. Although opioids affect gut motility there is little evidence that a single therapeutic dose given preoperatively increases the incidence of postoperative ileus.

Large doses of acepromazine are best avoided in horses that are to undergo colic surgery, at least until circulating volume is restored. This drug is a potent α_1-adrenergic blocker and may cause severe hypotension in a hypovolaemic horse that is compensating for the fluid loss by peripheral vasoconstriction. Acepromazine should help improve perfusion if the horse can be sufficiently hydrated, but in practice it is difficult to hydrate the horse adequately before anaesthesia.

Fluid administration

The circulating blood volume should, if possible, be restored before induction of anaesthesia; fluid that will stay in the circulation until surgery is well under way is required. Hypertonic saline (4 mL/kg of 7.5% solution) is ideal in these circumstances and is widely used. It draws fluid into the circulation and increases cardiac contractility and output. The effect can be dramatic and lasts well into the surgical period. The dose should not be repeated or sodium toxicity will occur. Only a small volume is required, some 2 L in a 500 kg horse, which can easily be given while the animal is prepared for surgery (Figure 8.2). Hypertonic saline infusion must be followed up later by isotonic

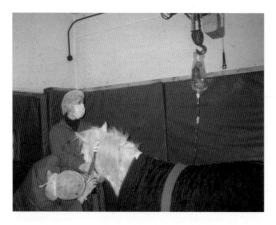

FIG 8.2 *Hypertonic saline is given immediately before induction of anaesthesia for emergency colic surgery. The pony is in the induction box ready for induction of anaesthesia.*

crystalloids to restore the ECF, but this can be given during surgery when the intestinal obstruction is relieved. Hydroxyethyl starches are also used to restore the circulation and have been highly successful. Doses of 10–30 mg/kg are generally used to support the circulation.

Alternatively, isotonic crystalloids can also be given before surgery, but larger volumes must be used. In this case a balance between restoration of the blood volume and complete rehydration must be achieved. If the whole of the calculated fluid deficit is given before anaesthesia a substantial proportion will diffuse into the lumen of the intestine before the obstruction can be relieved. Thus it will not only be lost from the circulation but will also make the surgery more difficult. If isotonic solutions are used, some 10–20 L can be given during preparation for surgery. As after hypertonic saline, the remaining ECF deficit is restored during surgery once the obstruction is relieved.

If possible, preparation for surgery, including clipping and surgical scrubbing, should be carried out before induction to keep anaesthesia time to a minimum. It is particularly important to minimise the time between induction of anaesthesia and relief of abdominal pressure.

ANAESTHESIA

The horse may have a grossly distended bowel, which will cause severe cardio-pulmonary embarrassment and may even rupture at induction. A stomach tube should be passed immediately before induction to empty the stomach, but unless it is very severe it is usually better to leave relief of more distal distension until surgery. The stomach tube can be left *in situ* but should be withdrawn above the cardiac sphincter, at least until the endotracheal tube is in place with the cuff inflated. Inhalation of stomach contents may be insidious and is often fatal.

The anaesthetic agents chosen for induction depend on personal preference: the best are usually those with which the anaesthetist is most familiar, as long as doses are adjusted appropriately. It is advisable to avoid large doses of either barbiturates or α_2 agonists, as these depress the cardiovascular system; long-term use of the α_2 agonists may also depress gut motility. The most common technique is to use α_2 agonists and ketamine (2 mg/kg) with or without diazepam (pages 34–37). Alternatively, combinations of guaiphenesin and thiopental or guaiphenesin and ketamine with or without small doses of xylazine or diazepam can be used (pages 37–39). The slow circulation in a sick horse with colic will lead to slow induction; the temptation to give further doses should be resisted. Halothane has been widely used for maintenance of anaesthesia, but isoflurane or sevoflurane are probably better.

The aims of anaesthetic maintenance are similar to those for any other procedure, except for the greater emphasis on fluid replacement and resolution of the effects of endotoxin. Progress is monitored using arterial blood pressure, pulse rate, mucous membrane colour, haematocrit and total protein measurements. Increasing haematocrit in the face of falling protein occurs in endotoxaemia and is difficult to treat. Plasma infusion (generally around 10 mL/kg) is indicated but rarely available for horses. Hypertonic saline, unless the maximum dose has already been given, is probably beneficial, but may transiently reduce cardiac output, which may be serious. Cardiac support with inotropes is essential (pages 80–81) to treat hypotension, as in healthy horses. Severely endotoxic horses may not respond. Horses undergoing colic surgery often need surprisingly little inhalation agent, and, unless they are endotoxic, may have good circulation once the volume deficit has been restored. It may be possible to keep anaesthesia at an apparently light plane; as long as movement is prevented, this is no cause for worry.

Respiratory depression may occur as in any horse. However, because IPPV depresses cardiac output by reducing venous return, hypotension may develop suddenly if IPPV is used in the face of hypovolaemia. A degree of hypercapnia is better tolerated than hypotension. IPPV may be essential until bowel distension is relieved in the severely bloated horse. Rapid surgical relief of distension is paramount in these circumstances.

Horses undergoing anaesthesia for colic may have acid–base imbalance, although a surprising number are relatively normal in this respect. It is impossible to assess acidosis or alkalosis unless blood gases can be measured. Treatment is often unnecessary, as restoration of blood flow to the renal and hepatic circulations in response to fluid therapy allows normal homoeostatic mechanisms to adjust the acid–base abnormalities without intervention. It is better to concentrate on fluid replacement if no means of blood gas measurement is available. If base deficit can be measured, bicarbonate can be given according to the formula:

$$\text{base excess} \times \text{body weight (kg)} \times 0.3 \text{ mEq.}$$

An 8.4% solution of sodium bicarbonate contains 1 mEq/mL. If bicarbonate is required ventilation must be increased because large quantities of carbon dioxide are produced according to the equation:

$$H^+ + HCO_3^- \Leftrightarrow H_2CO_3 \Leftrightarrow H_2O + CO_2$$

This excess carbon dioxide must be blown off, and in so doing will use up the carbon dioxide absorbent.

RECOVERY

If colic surgery has been successful, the horse is usually calm in the recovery period. If further analgesics or sedatives are required it often means that the problem has not been resolved. Postoperative monitoring and intravenous fluid therapy must continue once the horse is standing.

PREGNANCY AND CAESAREAN SECTION

PREGNANCY

Pregnancy induces a number of physiological changes, but it is only in later gestation that these have an impact on the course of anaesthesia in mares. Anaesthesia in pregnancy carries a risk of induced abortion. However, this is extremely rare, and if normal precautions about maintenance of cardiovascular and respiratory function are taken, anaesthesia in at least the first two trimesters carries no particular risk. There is no evidence that any of the anaesthetic drugs commonly used in horses causes fetal damage or loss, although xylazine increases uterine tone and low doses of detomidine are preferable. Towards the end of gestation the mechanical effects of a large, gravid uterus take effect. These are described below, as they apply equally to anaesthesia for caesarean section.

CAESAREAN SECTION

The parturient mare presented for caesarean section has similar needs to those of any acute case, with two additional considerations: first, the effect of the gravid uterus on the mare, and second the effect of anaesthetic drugs on the foal. A mare may exhibit abdominal pain, particularly if uterine torsion is the reason for surgery. She may also be exhausted and marginally dehydrated, but is unlikely to have the severe deficits seen in cases of intestinal obstruction.

Parturient animals require lower doses of anaesthetic agents than normal and should be dosed for their normal weight. Barbiturates are best avoided, and a single dose of xylazine followed by ketamine is often used successfully (pages 34–36). Alternatively, a combination of guaiphenesin (25–75 mg/kg) and ketamine (2 mg/kg) with or without small doses of xylazine (0.25–0.5 mg/kg) or diazepam (0.05–0.1 mg/kg) can be used. Other α_2 agonists can be used, but xylazine is the shortest acting and likely to have the least effect on the foal after birth. Any anaesthetic agent crosses the placenta, and those least depressant to the respiratory system should be used; barbiturates are the least satisfactory for this reason. Foals appear to be little affected by α_2 agonists and ketamine, and volatile-agent maintenance is satisfactory as the anaesthetic is rapidly blown off when the foal begins to breathe.

A major hazard of anaesthesia for caesarean section is compression of the vena cava when the mare is placed in dorsal recumbency (Figure 8.3). If the mare is placed symmetrically on her back a spectacular, sometimes fatal, hypotension may occur. The mare should be tilted off the midline as much as is compatible with surgery and arterial blood pressure should be monitored continuously before she is placed in dorsal recumbency, so that any position that causes hypotension is noticed and rectified as soon as it occurs. The weight

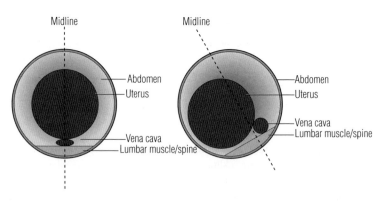

FIG 8.3 The pregnant mare should be tilted off the midline for caesarean section to reduce pressure from the gravid uterus on the vena cava. Once the foal has been delivered she can be repositioned more symmetrically.

of the gravid uterus also increases compression of the dependent lung, thereby reducing volatile anaesthetic uptake, and slightly higher vaporiser settings may be required to maintain anaesthesia until the foal is delivered.

A second anaesthetic machine for intubation and oxygen delivery, as well as an experienced clinician, should be available to resuscitate the foal. Once resuscitated, the foal should be kept as near the mare as possible but should not be loose with her until she is standing and no longer ataxic.

Anaesthesia is also used for dystocia and vaginal delivery. The same hazards apply to the mare, but gross physical manipulation of the mare's body makes the anaesthetist's job much more difficult. Careful monitoring of the cardiovascular and respiratory systems is essential so that the mare can be returned to a relaxed lateral position quickly if cardiovascular or respiratory function is seriously compromised.

HEAD AND NECK SURGERY

Special considerations for airway surgery are the risk of airway obstruction and the likelihood of vagal stimulation.

AIRWAY OBSTRUCTION

During surgery. 'Tie-back' surgery is normally carried out with an endotracheal tube in place and potential airway obstruction is a postoperative hazard. However, ventriculectomy is often carried out with the endotracheal tube removed. The horse is anaesthetised by any standard method and anaesthesia is maintained with inhalational agents while the site is prepared. The endotracheal tube is pulled rostrally immediately before access to the trachea is required. Surgery is either carried out very quickly and the tube repositioned, or anaesthesia is maintained with intravenous agents. 'Triple drip' (pages 41–43) is a suitable intravenous anaesthetic for this purpose, but anaesthesia must be relatively deep to prevent swallowing movements. The potential for blood clots to accumulate in and obstruct the trachea is significant, particularly if the laryngeal incision is closed after surgery. Airway obstruction is a potential complication of this operation.

Postoperative. Tie-back surgery carries a significant risk of apparently functional obstruction of the larynx. It is common practice to leave the endotracheal tube in place during recovery and remove it once the horse is standing. However, functional airway obstruction may not occur until up to 24 hours after surgery; these patients must be carefully monitored postoperatively. Any sign of respiratory stridor must be noted and equipment for emergency tracheotomy must be readily available. Perioperative NSAIDs may help to prevent oedema of the surgical site, and steroids (dexamethasone 2 mg/kg) may be given if there is any indication of stridor, with the risk of laminitis taken into account.

VAGAL STIMULATION

Laryngeal surgery of any kind carries the risk of vagal stimulation, leading to bradycardia or sinus arrest. Any neck surgery where the vagus may be manipulated or simply touched may initiate a similar response. The surest way to prevent a serious problem is to administer an anticholinergic (e.g. glycopyrrolate 0.005–0.01 mg/kg or atropine 0.005–0.02 mg/kg) before surgery begins. This may not block the response completely but it usually prevents cardiac arrest. Pre-surgical administration of glycopyrrolate also has the advantage that it can be given before any inotrope infusion has commenced, thereby avoiding the tachycardia seen when anticholinergics are given during the course of inotrope infusion (pages 29–30, 80–81). An alternative approach is to have a ready-loaded syringe of glycopyrrolate or atropine to hand, and to give it only if bradycardia develops. This approach is adequate if the horse is meticulously monitored, but cardiac arrest may occur with no preceding bradycardia.

Surgery of the neck anywhere in the vicinity of the vagus should be regarded as high risk; pre-surgical administration of an anticholinergic is not unwarranted in such cases.

GUTTURAL POUCH AND ETHMOID HAEMATOMA SURGERY

These procedures carry the added risk of severe haemorrhage. Guttural pouch surgery in particular may be required in an emergency to prevent further haemorrhage in a horse that has already lost a great deal of blood. The cardiovascular system should be carefully monitored. Direct arterial pressure is measured using an artery away from the head, usually the dorsal pedal (page 8 and Figure 5.3, page 90). Reliable venous access, with preferably more than one short large-gauge (10 or 12 swg) catheter must be secured. At least one site away from the head is advisable. Large volumes of IV fluid must be available; this is usually lactated Ringer's solution, although true plasma replacement solutions and, ideally, cross-matched blood should be available. Hypertonic saline is suitable for emergency restoration of circulation but is best used after haemostasis is secured. Equipment for packing off bleeding vessels must be readily available. It is important that there is no sudden surge in blood pressure, which may restart the haemorrhage. A smooth recovery is particularly important. The use of α_2 agonists should be limited, but although these initially cause hypertension, the arteriolar vasoconstriction responsible may be beneficial.

EYE SURGERY

Special considerations for eye surgery include the hazards of vagal stimulation and the problem of keeping the eye central and still during surgery.

THE OCULOCARDIAC REFLEX

Pressure on the eye causes vagal stimulation, leading to bradycardia and even sinus arrest. Any surgery around the eye may initiate this response, but it is most commonly seen with intraocular surgery or enucleation. The best way to prevent bradycardia is to administer an anticholinergic before surgery begins, as described above for airway surgery (page 192).

INTRAOCULAR PRESSURE

Raised intraocular pressure is highly undesirable when the globe is opened. This is particularly important during induction of anaesthesia before surgery to repair corneal lacerations or ruptured ulcers. It is also significant during any intraocular surgery and in the recovery period. Theoretically, drugs that increase intraocular pressure, particularly ketamine, should be avoided. However, when used in combination with sedatives and volatile agents, ketamine does not appear to cause any surgical problem and has been used successfully in numerous eye operations on horses. Coughing at intubation and vomiting are notorious for raising intraocular pressure, but because the horse does not do either of these they do not have to be considered.

Hypercapnia increases cerebral circulation, intracerebral pressure, and with it intraocular pressure, and should be avoided. It is worth using IPPV in all equine patients undergoing intraocular surgery, as even those that appear to breathe well tend to be hypercapnic.

EYE POSITION

Surgery of the globe requires that the eye be fixed, and for intraocular surgery it must also be central. Normally the eye is rotated forwards at a surgical depth of anaesthesia, making access for some operations difficult. Although the globe can be fixed with clamps it is more satisfactory if the reflexes are abolished.

Deep anaesthesia. Very deep volatile agent anaesthesia will fix the eye centrally, but this is not recommended as it is too close to death.

Neuromuscular blockade. Neuromuscular blockade with a non-depolarising agent, generally atracurium (pages 81–84), relaxes the oculomotor muscles and fixes the eye centrally. This is suitable for use in experienced hands for relatively prolonged surgery. However, the effect on the eye may not last as long as on limb muscles, and it may be necessary to keep the horse anaesthetised for some 30 minutes after surgery has been completed before the neuromuscular blockade can be reversed. Suxamethonium is contraindicated as this increases intraocular pressure.

Ketamine. Immediately after ketamine is injected IV during anaesthesia the eye becomes fixed and central. The effect usually lasts around 10 minutes after a dose of 0.2 mg/kg. For short surgical procedures on the eye this may be the most satisfactory method of providing good operating conditions.

Local anaesthesia. Retrobulbar block is used to provide intra- and postoperative analgesia as well as relaxed eye muscles in many species, and is equally applicable to the horse (see Figure 6.2b, page 112). It has the added advantage of abolishing the oculocardiac reflex once the block has taken effect.

RECOVERY

The eye and periorbital tissues are vulnerable to damage during a violent recovery. Raised intraocular pressures must be avoided after any ocular surgery to prevent wound breakdown and prolapse of intraocular structures. All attempts should be made to produce a calm recovery, but this cannot be guaranteed. Hoods with reinforced plastic globes to cover the eyes probably provide the best protection during recovery as long as they are well secured (Figure 8.4), but some horses do not tolerate these willingly.

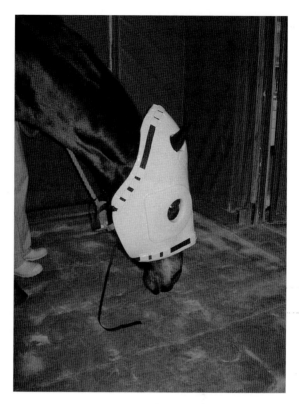

FIG 8.4   Hood to protect the eye during recovery from ocular surgery.

THE FOAL

The foal is relatively well developed when born, and in many respects responds to anaesthesia in the same way as an adult. Its smaller size reduces the risk of some of the problems seen in adults, such as myopathy, but there are other features, particularly in the newborn foal, that need particular attention.

In virtually all cases the foal should be kept with the dam as much as possible (Figure 8.5). This includes inducing anaesthesia with the dam present, and

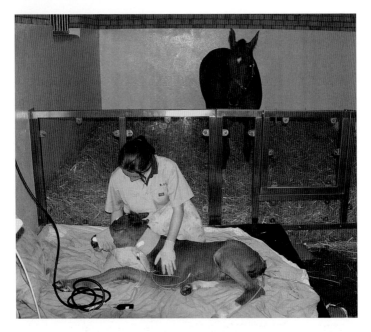

FIG 8.5   *Mare and foal will remain more calm if they are kept together as much as possible when the foal is conscious. (Photograph courtesy of Dr K Corley.)*

bringing the mare back to the foal, or taking the unconscious foal back to the mare for recovery. Both mare and foal remain calm when they are together, and induction and recovery are consequently smoother. It is usually necessary to sedate the mare before the foal is taken away for surgery after induction. Acepromazine may be sufficient but α_2 agonists are often required in addition.

TEMPERATURE

Although the foal's temperature regulation is good when conscious, most anaesthetics depress normal temperature regulation and its small size and low body fat mean that the foal loses heat much more rapidly than the adult. Use of 'bubble wrap' or space blankets, heated pads, hot air blowers (Figure 8.6) and warmed intravenous and irrigating fluids helps to maintain body temperature. It is easier to prevent heat loss than to warm a cold animal, and care should be taken throughout anaesthesia to prevent hypothermia.

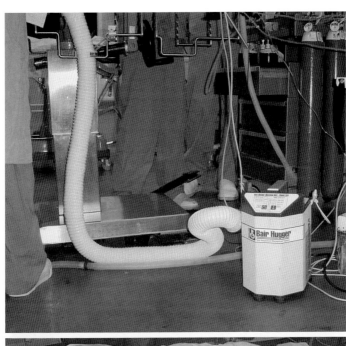

A

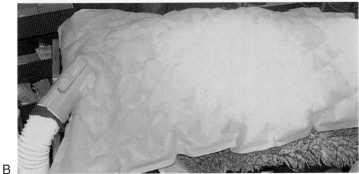

B

FIG 8.6   Normal body temperature should be maintained during anaesthesia. This is effectively accomplished with a commercially available heater which (A) blows warm air through wide-bore tubing into (B) a double-sided blanket perforated on one side which is placed over the anaesthetized foal.

Hypothermia will delay recovery as drug metabolism is slowed; shivering during rewarming increases oxygen consumption.

ENERGY AND METABOLISM

The newborn foal maintains blood glucose well if starved, but the fat store is very limited and foals may become hypoglycaemic during or after anaesthesia; dextrose should therefore be administered with electrolyte solutions during anaesthesia. Preoperative starvation be kept to a minimum. Regurgitation during anaesthesia is uncommon in foals, and newborns do not need to be starved at all.

STRESS

Foals tolerate anaesthesia and surgery well, but any stress is likely to cause gastric ulceration. This is best prevented by the administration of H_2 antagonists (e.g. cimetidine 2 mg/kg orally, IV or IM qid, or ranitidine 0.5 mg/kg bid orally) and demulcents (e.g. sucralfate 2 mg/kg tid orally) from the day of surgery for a few days postoperatively. Omeprazole is the only gastric protectant licensed for equine use, but there is less experience of its use in association with anaesthesia.

THE CARDIORESPIRATORY SYSTEM

The newborn foal's circulation has recently adjusted from fetal to adult configuration. The ductus arteriosus and foramen ovale are not completely sealed in the first few days of life, and an increase in pulmonary resistance may cause blood flow to revert to the fetal configuration, causing profound hypoxaemia. Particular care should be taken to prevent hypoxia and acidosis, which increase pulmonary vascular resistance. Incomplete expansion of the lungs and patchy atelectasis may be present, particularly in the premature foal, leading to hypoxaemia, which can only be improved by the provision of very high inspired oxygen concentrations.

The newborn foal's response to hypoxia and hypercapnia is immature. When anaesthetised with respiratory depressant anaesthetic drugs, respiratory depression may be even more severe than in the adult. Oxygen-enriched gases must be used and IPPV may be necessary even for relatively short procedures.

The newborn foal is dependent on heart rate to maintain cardiac output. Drugs that cause bradycardia and increased afterload (α_2 agonists) or reduce preload must be used with care.

PHARMACOKINETICS

Uptake and elimination of injected drugs differ from the adult in a number of ways. Immature animals have underdeveloped mechanisms for renal and hepatic clearance of drugs. Low body fat and plasma albumin also affect the pharmacokinetics. The overall result is that the foal requires smaller doses of protein-bound drugs such as barbiturates, but may be resistant to the nonprotein-bound agents such as ketamine. Drugs that are normally redistributed to fat or are cleared by liver and kidney (most injectable sedatives and anaesthetics) may have a longer duration of action.

SEDATION AND PREMEDICATION

A number of minor procedures can be performed on sedated foals and most agents or combinations used for sedation can also be used for premedication (see Chapter 2). Foals lie down more readily than adults and sedation may often induce recumbency (see Figure 2.5). Once they are past the neonatal stage (when benzodiazepines alone are adequate) healthy foals can be safely sedated with xylazine (1 mg/kg) and their response is similar to that in the adult. Detomidine has also been widely used in the foal at doses of 0.01–0.02 mg/kg, similar to the adult. Romifidine (0.05–0.1 mg/kg) has a similar effect. The addition of butorphanol (0.02–0.04 mg/kg) produces excellent sedation and analgesia that allows many minor procedures such as radiography, cast changes and aspirations to be performed. However, the α_2 agonists have dramatic cardiovascular effects and should be used very carefully with volatile-agent anaesthesia in very young foals.

Phenothiazine sedation has a similar mild effect in foals to that in adults, and generally requires supplementation with an opioid to allow diagnostic procedures to be performed. It should not be used in the hypovolaemic foal as it may cause severe hypotension. It may be useful for premedication before inhalation induction and to smooth recovery.

Benzodiazepines such as diazepam and midazolam (0.1–0.25 mg/kg) are used both alone and in combination with opioids such as butorphanol (0.02 mg/kg) for sedation and premedication. Diazepam is not water soluble and may cause pain on injection, but solutions in fat emulsion are less irritant. Midazolam is water soluble and shorter acting. The benzodiazepines are particularly suitable for premedication before nasal intubation for gaseous induction and before ketamine anaesthesia. In the newborn foal, diazepam or midazolam on its own usually produces enough sedation for many procedures.

GENERAL ANAESTHESIA

Induction of anaesthesia in healthy newborn foals can be accomplished by inhalation of a volatile agent (halothane, isoflurane and sevoflurane have all been used). Induction is generally smooth and recovery rapid. Most newborn foals tolerate this well and premedication is not necessary. A purpose-built mask or a nasal tube can be used to administer the gas. Use of a nasal tube allows a smooth transition from induction to endotracheal intubation as the endotracheal tube can be inserted without removing the nasal tube. During induction the other nostril should be gently closed by the person restraining the head. The mare should be kept with the foal until it is unconscious.

Inhalation induction appears to be associated with a risk of cardiac arrest. This problem is most obvious in sick foals and may be related to the effects of electrolyte imbalance, acidosis and high circulating catecholamines. An alternative that appears to be safer is premedication with diazepam (0.2 mg/kg) or midazolam (0.2 mg/kg) immediately before induction of anaesthesia with ketamine (2 mg/kg). The benzodiazepine can be mixed in the syringe with the ketamine and both administered together. Again, the dam should remain with the foal until it is unconscious. Older foals (up to around 3 months) can also be safely anaesthetised this way.

Older foals (3–6 months) can be sedated with an α_2 agonist (xylazine 0.5 mg/kg, detomidine 0.01 mg/kg or romifidine 0.05 mg/kg) and butorphanol (0.02 mg/kg) and anaesthetised with ketamine (2 mg/kg IV). Premedication with IV midazolam (0.2 mg/kg) or diazepam (0.25 mg/kg) is also acceptable in older foals before ketamine induction in cases where α_2 agonists are considered undesirable. Methadone or morphine (0.1 mg/kg) can be substituted for the butorphanol. Foals over about 6 months can be treated like adults.

It is better to avoid barbiturates in the very young foal, as recovery may be prolonged and respiratory depression more pronounced. Foals over 2–3 months respond to barbiturates more like adults.

Anaesthesia for major surgery is most commonly maintained with a volatile agent. Anaesthetic breathing circuits, generally circle systems, used for dogs and humans are suitable for young foals up to around 100–120 kg (Figure 8.7). Volatile agent anaesthesia in the foal is similar to that in the adult, but cardiovascular and respiratory depression may be marked in the spontaneously

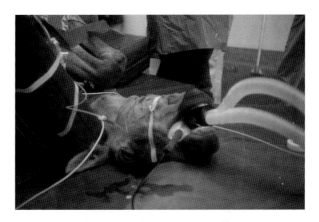

FIG 8.7a Anaesthetic equipment suitable for large dogs or human anaesthesia is used in young foals.

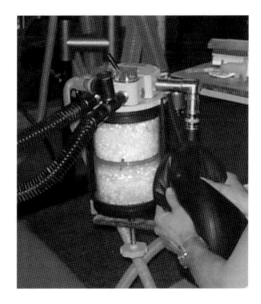

FIG 8.7b This equipment, such as the circle system shown here, can also be used for manual ventilation if required.

breathing foal. Severe respiratory acidosis and hypotension may develop rapidly. Foals respond well to IPPV and inotropic support with dobutamine or dopamine at doses used in adults (pages 80–81). Blood pressure is lower in foals than in adult horses, and a mean pressure not less than 60 mmHg is a suitable goal. Intravenous fluid infusion should be given for cardiac support and should include 5% dextrose to maintain normoglycaemia, as discussed above.

Recovery from anaesthesia is much easier to manage in foals than in adults, as they are small enough to control and assist. If the dam is calm, it may help to allow the foal to recover in her presence.

SPECIFIC CONDITIONS

Anaesthesia of the newborn foal is commonly required for repair of ruptured bladder, colic (often due to a congenital abnormality), orthopaedic repair, or treatment of a head injury. Management of these conditions is similar to that which would be employed in an adult or another species, but each condition has a number of aspects in the foal that require special mention.

Ruptured bladder and uroperitoneum

These cases are hypovolaemic, have cardiorespiratory embarrassment due to a distended abdomen, and cardiac dysrhythmias as a result of hyperkalaemia, hyponatraemia and uraemia.

Circulating blood volume should be restored before induction of anaesthesia; isotonic saline helps to restore the sodium and chloride deficit. Further saline may be needed to return values to normal after the circulatory deficit has been replaced. Hyperkalaemia can be treated with insulin and glucose (0.1 IU/kg insulin and 0.5 mg/kg dextrose in 500 mL saline). Other ionic deficits, such as calcium, may require treatment.

The urine should be drained from the abdomen to relieve abdominal distension before induction of anaesthesia. IPPV will help to ensure adequate ventilation during surgery, at least until any remaining abdominal distension has been relieved.

Hyperkalaemia and uraemia may cause ventricular dysrhythmias. Anaesthesia may precipitate dysrhythmias and cardiac insufficiency, and any dysrhyth-mogenic drugs such as the α_2 agonists should be avoided. Induction with benzodiazepine–ketamine appears well tolerated, although the very sick foal may be intubated and given a volatile agent without any induction agent. Anaesthesia is best maintained with a volatile agent, using isoflurane or sevoflurane in preference to halothane, as they are less dysrhythmogenic. Atropine, adrenaline (epinephrine) and lidocaine (pages 132–133) should be available to treat any dysrhythmias that occur during anaesthesia.

Colic
Anaesthetic management of the foal with gastrointestinal obstruction is similar to that in the adult. The foal is small enough that hetastarch or gelatine plasma replacers can be used to restore the circulating blood volume before anaesthesia. Fluid therapy during anaesthesia should include some dextrose, as discussed above. Careful monitoring of fluid input and urine output is particularly valuable in the foal, where there is less margin for error in the volume transfused.

Respiratory and circulatory embarrassment due to abdominal distension may be a serious problem and the aim should be to support the circulation, provide IPPV and decompress the intestine as soon as possible.

Orthopaedic surgery
Anaesthesia for orthopaedic surgery in the foal is managed in a similar manner to that in the adult. The animal is generally otherwise healthy and the main consideration is provision of good pre- and postoperative analgesia. Premedication with an opioid such as morphine, methadone or butorphanol is effective; postoperative analgesia can be improved with additional flunixin (1.0 mg/kg) given during surgery. Flunixin may increase the likelihood of gastric ulceration, and postoperative administration of demulcents and H_2 blockers or omeprazole is essential.

Head injury
Head injury is a more common presentation for emergency surgery in foals than in adults, but the same general principles apply. Increased intracranial pressure is to be avoided, hence anything that increases cerebral blood flow is contraindicated. In theory, ketamine, volatile agents, hypercapnia, and large volumes of intravenous electrolyte and dextrose fluids should be avoided. Barbiturates, which reduce intracranial pressure and metabolism, are drugs of choice and diuretics, including furosemide and mannitol, can be used to decrease cerebral oedema.

In practice, ventilation should always be controlled in order to prevent hypercapnia or even to produce slight hypocapnia. Hypoxaemia is prevented with high inspired oxygen if necessary. Fluid therapy should be sufficient to maintain adequate circulation, but overinfusion must be avoided. In spite of the theory, ketamine can be used in small doses as well as barbiturates, and volatile agents are used quite successfully in spite of the effect on cerebral blood flow. Isoflurane or sevoflurane are preferable to halothane as the effect is less marked and more easily controlled by hyperventilation. Benzodiazepine premedication is indicated as it decreases cerebral blood flow and increases the seizure threshold.

HYPERKALAEMIC PERIODIC PARALYSIS (HYPP)

HYPP is caused by an inherited genetic defect of the sodium channel in muscle. The channels are leaky, leading to muscle tremor and paralysis when circulating potassium is high. This may be triggered by stress, or by diets high in potassium. The condition is seen only in Quarter horses who are descendants of a prolific stallion, 'Impressive'. The condition is rare, particularly outside the USA, but necessitates special consideration if anaesthesia is required. There is a genetic test to detect affected animals: this is worthwhile if 'Impressive' may be in the horse's ancestry.

For elective procedures the horse can be treated with oral acetazolamide for 2 days before surgery (2 mg bid). It should also be kept on a low-potassium diet, have regular exercise, small frequent meals, and not be stressed. For anaesthesia, it should not be fasted and should not be given potassium-containing fluids, including potassium salts of any drug (e.g. penicillin). The procedure should be as smooth and stress free as possible, so good sedation and a quiet induction are more important than the precise drugs used. Careful monitoring of the ECG, blood gases and pH, as well as ventilation to prevent acidosis, are required. All treatment drugs must be available during anaesthesia, should signs develop, particularly ECG abnormalities, sweating and muscle tremor. Treatment includes calcium (20% calcium gluconate 0.2–0.4 mL/kg), dextrose (5%, 2–6 mL/kg), sodium bicarbonate (1–2 mEq/kg), insulin (0.05 IU/kg) and furosemide (0.4 mg/kg); in an emergency injectable acetazolamide (0.5 mg/kg IV) may also be useful.

GLYCOGEN STORAGE DISEASE

Glycogen storage disease is another rare, inherited genetic defect that may cause problems in anaesthesia. It is seen in some lines of warmblood dressage horses, but is impossible to diagnose with certainty except by genetic typing. Anaesthesia may trigger a severe episode of generalised rhabdomyolysis, which is likely to be fatal. If the genetic predisposition is suspected the horse should be kept on a high-lipid, low-carbohydrate diet for as long as possible prior to surgery. Such special diets are now commercially available from some specialist equine feed compounders. If there is no time for a preparatory diet, preoperative oral dantrolene (1–4 mg/kg) may prevent the development of myopathy and is the best line of prevention. Injectable dantrolene is very expensive. No particular anaesthetic techniques have been found to be of particular benefit, but every effort should be made to prevent muscle ischaemia during anaesthesia, as this is likely to increase the risk of myopathy. If postoperative myopathy does occur, treatment is symptomatic as already described in Chapter 7 (pages 146–148). If the horse is severely affected and recumbent the prognosis should be guarded.

DONKEYS

In many respects donkeys, mules and tame zebras respond to sedation and general anaesthesia in the same way as domestic horses and ponies. However, a few notable differences deserve special mention. It is more difficult to estimate weight, and tapes and formulae tend to underestimate (pages 10–11).

SPECIFIC DRUG EFFECTS

The effect of α_2 agonists is somewhat variable in donkeys and many are quite resistant. It is best to give the dose that would be required in a horse and give an additional quarter to half the dose if the effect of the first is inadequate.

Immobilon (neuroleptic combination of etorphine and acepromazine, see pages 52–53) is contraindicated in donkeys. A high incidence of post-recovery excitement occurs in spite of judicious use of antagonists.

INTUBATION

Donkeys are more difficult to intubate than horses. The larynx and trachea are proportionately smaller, the larynx is softer and the epiglottis more easily displaced. A smaller tube than anticipated should be used, the neck should be fully extended, and intubation should be as gentle as possible. Nasal intubation is sometimes easier.

RECOVERY

Donkeys are far more sensible in recovery than horses. They are easier to assist as they are smaller, but this is often unnecessary as they remain calm, usually in sternal recumbency, until they are able to stand without ataxia.

WILD AND AGGRESSIVE HORSES

There are occasions when an unhandled or really aggressive domestic horse must be caught, sedated and anaesthetised. There is a serious risk that the horse may injure itself or the handlers. The high level of excitement means that sedative drugs are not as effective as usual and the inevitably high circulating catecholamines enhance the risk of ventricular dysrhythmias.

If IM injections are feasible, a combination of detomidine (0.03 mg/kg), butorphanol (0.02 mg/kg) and acepromazine (0.03 mg/kg) will often calm the horse sufficiently to allow IV catheterisation and normal management. It is essential that the horse be given at least 30 minutes completely undisturbed after injection for this to be effective. This combination has more chance of success than α_2 agonists alone.

If the horse cannot be injected, sublingual detomidine (0.03–0.04 mg/kg) may calm it sufficiently for handling. This can be either squirted under the tongue with a syringe or given in a sugar lump or chewy sweet, so that it is not swallowed immediately. The drug must be absorbed through the mucous membrane, as it is not effective if swallowed.

If the horse is completely unhandleable it may be possible to get it to eat something sticky laced with detomidine. Alternatively, an old method using oral chloral hydrate is worth a try. Most horses will not drink water with chloral hydrate in it as it is very pungent, but may eat dry crystals mixed with molassed grain feed; 100 mg/kg should be given.

Once the horse is caught and handled it can be treated as normal as far as anaesthetic drugs are concerned. However, it must be appreciated that it may have been treated with high doses of sedative agents, and great care must be taken to assure good cardiovascular and respiratory function.

Exotic wild equidae such as Prewalski's horses do not respond to sedation in the same way as domestic horses. In these, and in the occasional untouched domestic horse, darting with etorphine is the most reliable to ensure restraint and capture. In this instance, assistance from a veterinarian with the necessary skills, dart gun and licence is necessary.

Further reading

Clutton RE (1997) Remote intramuscular injection in unmanageable horses. *In Practice* **19**: 316–319.

Corley KTT (2004) Fluid therapy. In: Bertone JJ and Horsepool LJI (eds) *Equine Clinical Pharmacology.* WB Saunders, London, Chapter 17, 327–364.

Edwards JGT, Newton JR, Ramzan PHL, et al (2003) The efficacy of dantrolene sodium in controlling exertional rhabdomyolysis in the Thoroughbred racehorse. *Equine Veterinary Journal* **35**: 707–711.

Hubbell JA, Hinchcliff KW, Schmall LM, et al (2000) Anesthetic, cardiorespiratory, and metabolic effects of four intravenous anesthetic regimens induced in horses immediately after maximal exercise. *American Journal of Veterinary Research* **61**: 1545–1552.

Klein L (1985) Anesthesia for neonatal foals. *Veterinary Clinics of North America. Equine Practice* **1**: 77–89.

Matthews NS, Taylor TS & Hartsfield S (1997) Anaesthesia of donkeys and mules. *Equine Veterinary Education* **9**: 198–202.

McKenzie EC, Valberg SJ, Godden SM, et al (2004) Effect of oral administration of dantrolene sodium on serum creatine kinase activity after exercise in horses with recurrent exertional rhabdomyolysis. *American Journal of Veterinary Research* **65**: 74–79.

Muir WW and Hubbell JAE (1991) *Muir and Hubbell's Equine Anaesthesia: Monitoring and Emergency Therapy.* Mosby Year Book, St Louis.

Thurmon JC, Tranquilli WJ and Benson GJ (1996) *Lumb and Jones' Veterinary Anaesthesia,* 3rd edn. Williams & Wilkins, Baltimore.

Tranquilli WJ and Thurmon JC (1990) Management of anesthesia in the foal. *Veterinary Clinics of North America, Equine Practice* **6**: 651–663.

APPENDIX – EUROPEAN LAW AND THE HORSE AS A FOOD ANIMAL

1) Drugs with market authorization. Medicinal products with market authorization for use in horses destined for human consumption may be used in any horse according to the manufacturer's directions.

2) Drugs in Annex II*. In addition, using the 'cascade', products in 'Annex II' may be used in any horse, as long as the statutory withdrawal period (currently 28 days) is allowed. Annex II contains drugs deemed safe enough not to require a maximum residue limit (MRL), and may be used in food animals, via the cascade, without specific market authorisation for the species. Annex II includes several anaesthetic and related drugs, including, for example, isoflurane, ketamine, detomidine and romifidine. The status of medicinal products that have been assessed for MRL requirement can be found on the European Medicines Agency (EMEA) website. Veterinary medicines are covered at: *http://www.emea.eu.int/index/indexv1.htm*. The MRL section of this webpage contains summary assessments of each drug; its allocation to Annex II or otherwise is included in the final conclusions.

3) The positive list for horses. The 'positive list' of drugs for horses is a list of drugs that are necessary for normal veterinary treatment of horses, but do not have market authorization for the species, nor are in Annex II. The list is currently under consideration by the European Commission. If approved, these drugs may be used in horses intended for human consumption as long as a 6-month withdrawal period is allowed. All such drug use must be recorded in the horse's passport.

Anaesthetic-related drugs on the proposed positive list:

Sedation/premedication (and antagonism)/injectable anaesthesia
    Acepromazine
    Atipamezole
    Diazepam

*Annex II of Council Regulation (EEC) No. 2377/90

Midazolam
Naloxone
Propofol
Sarmazenil
Tiletamine
Zolazepam
For treatment of cardiovascular or respiratory depression
Dobutamine
Dopamine
Ephedrine
Glycopyrrolate
Noradrenaline (norepinephrine)
Analgesia
Buprenorphine
Fentanyl
Morphine
Pethidine
Muscle relaxation
Atracurium
Edrophonium
Guaiphenesin
Inhalation anaesthesia
Sevoflurane
Local anaesthesia
Bupivacaine
Oxybuprocaine
Prilocaine

INDEX

Drug combinations for sedation and premedication

Sedative combination	Dose for sedation	Dose for premedication
Acepromazine Xylazine	0.02–0.05 mg/kg 0.5–0.6 mg/kg	0.03–0.04 mg/kg 1.0 mg/kg
Acepromazine Detomidine	0.03–0.04 mg/kg 0.01 mg/kg	0.03–0.04 mg/kg 0.01–0.02 mg/kg
Acepromazine Romifidine	0.03–0.04 mg/kg 0.05 mg/kg	0.03–0.04 mg/kg 0.1 mg/kg
Acepromazine Butorphanol	0.02–0.05 mg/kg 0.02–0.04 mg/kg	0.03–0.05 mg/kg 0.02 mg/kg
Acepromazine Methadone	0.05–0.1 mg/kg 0.1 mg/kg	0.03–0.04 mg/kg 0.1 mg/kg
Xylazine Butorphanol	0.5–1.0 mg/kg 0.02 mg/kg	0.5–1.0 mg/kg 0.01–0.02 mg/kg.